# Monographs on Endocrinology



Volume 22

D.T. Krieger

# Cushing's Syndrome

With 27 Figures in 44 Separate Illustrations, Some in Color, and 24 Tables

Springer-Verlag
Berlin Heidelberg NewYork 1982

Dorothy T. Krieger, M. D.

Professor of Medicine
Director, Division of Endocrinology
The Mount Sinai Medical Center
One Gustave L. Levy Place
New York, N. Y. 10029/USA

Library of Congress Cataloging in Publication Data.
Krieger, Dorothy T. 1927-. Cushing's syndrome.
(Monographs on endocrinology; v. 22) Includes bibliographical
references and index. 1. Cushing's syndrome. I. Title. II. Series.
RC659.K74 616.4'5 81-9287
ISBN-13: 978-3-642-81661-1 e-ISBN-13: 978-3-642-81659-8
DOI: 10.1007/978-3-642-81659-8


Softcover reprint of the hardcover 1st edition 1982



2125/3020 543210

# Foreword

The unraveling of our knowledge of the functions of the adrenal gland constitutes one exciting development of modern medicine and biochemistry. We owe these advances to the felicitous cooperative efforts of the clinical investigator and the biochemist. Three centuries elapsed between the first recorded anatomical description of the adrenals and the demonstration by Dr. Addison in the mid-nineteenth century of the fatal results of the destruction of these glands by disease. It became evident from this observation that the adrenals secreted a "factor" or "factors" essential to life. It took approximately 90 years to isolate this elusive vital factor – cortisone – from beef adrenal cortices, independently by both Reichstein and his co-workers in Basle and Kendall and his group in the United States and another 10–15 years before it became more generally available for experimental and clinical use.

It is perhaps difficult to believe that as recently as 35–40 years ago, before cortisone and cortisol were clinically available, the surgical removal of a benign adrenal cortical tumor in patients with Cushing's syndrome was associated with a prohibitive postoperative mortality rate. Within 12–36 h after operation, most of such patients developed an intractable state of shock, which was not manifested by significant electrolyte abnormalities or hypoglycemia and was unresponsive to the usual treatment for shock plus the generous use of salt-retaining hormone. This critical situation was completely corrected when the glucogenic steroids came into use. It was realized that with the removal of the tumor such patients were rendered severely hypocortisolemic, since the function of the contralateral adrenal had been suppressed by the increased level of glucogenic steroid secreted by the tumor. This situation was often not so critical following the removal of a malignant adrenal cortical tumor, only because functioning metastases had already occurred prior to operation.

While the management of patients with Cushing's syndrome became clear and well defined, the problem of the pathogenesis and management of Cushing's disease (nontumorous adrenal cortical hypercortisolism) is considerably more complicated. In this excellent volume by Dr. Krieger, this problem and others related to adrenal cortical hyperfunction are thoroughly and thoughtfully addressed. Since the initial description of this disease by Dr. Cushing in 1912 and his more advanced and summarized studies in 1932, the increase in biochemical and physiological information concerning the neuroendocrinological factors and pathways involved in the eventual increase in the pituitary and ectopic secretion of ACTH have advanced considerably. Similarly, more options have become available in the clinical management of this illness. Today, bilateral adrenalectomy is certainly a feasible form of therapy, but hardly the most desirable except under very special and critical circumstances.

The mass of new information concerning the pathogenesis and management of Cushing's disease makes this a timely period to attempt to bring order into this diverse and complicated problem. Dr. Krieger, with her extensive experimental and clinical experience in this field, is particularly suited to focus directly on the various current problems and theses and to provide a coherent bridge to further developments.

Dr. Louis J. Soffer,
Emeritus Clinical Professor,
Mount Sinai School of Medicine,
New York, NY 10029, USA

# Contents

**Chapter 1. Brief Introduction to Cushing's Syndrome and Disease** . . . . . 1

References . . . . . . . . . . . . . . . . . . . . . . . . . 4

**Chapter 2. Physiology of Regulation of ACTH Secretion** . . . . . . . . . . 5

A. Chemistry of ACTH . . . . . . . . . . . . . . . . . . . . 5

B. Histology . . . . . . . . . . . . . . . . . . . . . . . . 6

C. Physiology of ACTH Secretion . . . . . . . . . . . . . . . . 8

I. Corticotropin-Releasing Factor . . . . . . . . . . . . . . 9

II. Neurotransmitter Regulation of ACTH Release . . . . . . . . 10

III. Neuroanatomical Pathways Involved in ACTH Release . . . . . 11

IV. Feedback Regulation of ACTH . . . . . . . . . . . . . . . 12

V. Circadian Periodicity . . . . . . . . . . . . . . . . . . 14

VI. Newer Aspects of Release of ACTH and Related Peptides . . . . . . . . . . . . . . . . . . . . 16

References . . . . . . . . . . . . . . . . . . . . . . . . . 18

**Chapter 3. ACTH Action** . . . . . . . . . . . . . . . . . . . 23

A. Structure-Function Relationships . . . . . . . . . . . . . . . 23

B. Effect on Adrenal Size, Morphology, and Growth . . . . . . . . . . 24

C. Mechanism of ACTH Action of Steroidogenesis . . . . . . . . . . . 25

D. Effect of ACTH on Aldosterone Secretion . . . . . . . . . . . . . 26

E. Dynamics of ACTH Secretion . . . . . . . . . . . . . . . . . 26

F. Extra-adrenal Metabolic Actions of ACTH . . . . . . . . . . . . 28

G. Behavioral Effects of ACTH . . . . . . . . . . . . . . . . . 29

References . . . . . . . . . . . . . . . . . . . . . . . . . 30

**Chapter 4. Actions of Adrenocortical Hormones** . . . . . . . . . . . . . 33

A. Pathways of Corticosteroid Biosynthesis . . . . . . . . . . . . . 35

B. Mechanism of Glucocorticoid Action . . . . . . . . . . . . . . . 35

References . . . . . . . . . . . . . . . . . . . . . . . . . 39

**Chapter 5. The Nature of ACTH-Related Peptides in Cushing's Disease and Syndrome** . . . . . . . . . . . . . . . . . . . . . . . 40

References . . . . . . . . . . . . . . . . . . . . . . . . . 42

**Chapter 6. Clinical Manifestations of Cushing's Disease and Cushing's Syndrome** . . . 44

A. Cushing's Disease . . . 44
I. Pathogenesis . . . 44
II. Signs and Symptoms . . . 47
III. Cushing's Disease and Pregnancy . . . 53
IV. Cushing's Syndrome and Disease in Children . . . 53
V. Familial Cushing's Syndrome . . . 54
VI. Nelson's Syndrome . . . 54
VII. Adrenal Pathology . . . 57
VIII. Animal Models of Cushing's Disease . . . 57
IX. Variant of Micronodular Hyperplasia . . . 57

B. Adrenal Tumors . . . 58

C. "Primary" Pituitary Tumor . . . 59

D. Ectopic ACTH Production . . . 60

E. Differential Diagnosis of Cushing's Disease and Syndrome . . . 64

References . . . 67

**Chapter 7. Laboratory Diagnosis of Cushing's Disease and Syndrome** . . . 73

A. Measurement of Basal Corticosteroid Production . . . 75
I. Nature of Steroids in Blood and Urine . . . 75
II. Plasma Corticosteroid Concentrations . . . 77
III. Circadian Variation of Plasma Corticosteroid Concentrations . . 78
IV. Other Plasma Steroids . . . 80
V. Urine Corticosteroid Concentrations . . . 80
VI. Urinary 17-Ketosteroids . . . 81
VII. Cortisol Production Rates . . . 82

B. Plasma ACTH Concentrations . . . 82

C. ACTH-Related Peptides: Lipotropin, Endorphin, and MSH . . . 85

D. Tests Involving Pituitary-Adrenal Stimulation and Suppression . . . 88
I. Adrenal Response to Exogenous ACTH Administration . . . 88
II. Response to Vasopressin . . . 88
III. Metyrapone Test: Response to Decrease in Cortisol Feedback . . 89
IV. Insulin Tolerance Test . . . 90
V. Dexamethasone Suppression Test . . . 91
VI. Multiple-Dose Dexamethasone Suppression Test . . . 92
VII. Multiple High-Dose Suppression Test . . . 92

E. Response to Hypothalamic-Releasing Hormones . . . 94
I. Thyrotropin-Releasing Hormone . . . 94
II. Gonadotropin-Releasing Hormone . . . 94
III. Somatostatin . . . 95
IV. Growth Hormone Responses . . . 95
V. Prolactin . . . 95
VI. Thyroid Hormones . . . 96
VII. Testosterone . . . 96

VIII. Nonspecific Diagnostic Determinations . . . . . . . . . . . . . 96
F. Usefulness of Hormonal Tests in Differential Diagnosis . . . . . . . . 97
G. Venous Catheterization for Ectopic ACTH-Producing Tumor Localization 103
H. Pituitary X-Ray Localization . . . . . . . . . . . . . . . . . . . . 104
J. Adrenal Localization . . . . . . . . . . . . . . . . . . . . . . . . 105
I. X-Ray Visualization . . . . . . . . . . . . . . . . . . . . 105
II. Radioscanning . . . . . . . . . . . . . . . . . . . . . . 107
III. Ultrasonography . . . . . . . . . . . . . . . . . . . . . 108
IV. Computerized Tomography . . . . . . . . . . . . . . . . . 108
V. Angiography . . . . . . . . . . . . . . . . . . . . . . . 112
References . . . . . . . . . . . . . . . . . . . . . . . . . . . . . 113

**Chapter 8. Treatment of Cushing's Disease and Syndrome** . . . . . . . . . 119

A. Adrenal Adenoma . . . . . . . . . . . . . . . . . . . . . . . . . 119
B. Adrenocortical Carcinoma . . . . . . . . . . . . . . . . . . . . . 119
I. o,p'DDD (Lysodren, Mitotane) . . . . . . . . . . . . . . . 119
II. Aminoglutethimide . . . . . . . . . . . . . . . . . . . . 120
C. Ectopic ACTH-Producing Tumors . . . . . . . . . . . . . . . . . 120
D. Cushing's Disease . . . . . . . . . . . . . . . . . . . . . . . . 121
I. Adrenal Surgery . . . . . . . . . . . . . . . . . . . . . 122
II. Adrenal-Directed Pharmacological Therapy . . . . . . . . . 124
III. Pituitary Irradiation and Surgery . . . . . . . . . . . . . . 126
IV. Medical Treatment . . . . . . . . . . . . . . . . . . . . 131
References . . . . . . . . . . . . . . . . . . . . . . . . . . . . . 135

**Subject Index** . . . . . . . . . . . . . . . . . . . . . . . . . . 139

*Chapter 1*

# Brief Introduction to Cushing's Syndrome and Disease

Harvey Cushing's classic monograph, *The Basophil Adenomas of the Pituitary Body and Their Clinical Manifestations,* was published in 1932. However, he first described a patient with this disease in 1912, characterizing it as a peculiar polyglandular syndrome including painful obesity, hypertrichosis, and amenorrhea, with overdevelopment of secondary sexual characteristics. At that time, he noted that, "whether these symptoms were chiefly attributable to disordered pituitary, adrenal, pineal or ovarian influences was uncertain." Cushing's description of the disease included all of those physical features which today we recognize as being classical. It is also of interest that a follow-up of the patient over a period of 22 years following the onset of the disease noted her to be in "reasonably good health, though some of the stigmata of her malady still persist."

Since 1932, we have become aware of diverse pathological etiologies of hypercorticism or Cushing's syndrome, reserving the term "Cushing's disease" for those cases of adrenal hyperfunction or hyperplasia with or without demonstrable small or large pituitary adenomata (Table 1.1).

In the case of adrenal or ectopic adrenocorticotropic hormone-producing tumors, there is no difficulty in relating the pathological process present to the clinical manifestations of adrenal cortical hyperfunction. However, the pathogenetic factors that lead to ectopic production of adrenocorticotropic hormone (ACTH), and the chemical nature of the ACTH secreted under such circumstances, remain fascinating subjects for investigation. Since the initial description of Cushing's disease, its etiology has been characterized as being secondary to pathology of either the pituitary, the adrenals, or the hypothalamus. In the introduction to his 1932 monograph, Cushing made some prescient statements which can still be appreciated by today's endocrinologists.

**Table 1.1.** Pathological findings in Cushing's syndrome

| | |
|---|---|
| Adrenal hyperplasia[a] | (ca. 50%–70%) |
| Pituitary adenoma[b] | |
| Pre-adrex | (ca. 10%) |
| Post-adrex | (ca. 15%–20%) |
| Nodular adrenal hyperplasia | Rare |
| Adrenal adenoma / Adrenal carcinoma | (ca. 20%–30%) |
| Ectopic tumors | (ca. 10%) |

[a] No evidence of sellar enlargement on routine X-ray.
[b] Enlarged sella evident on routine sellar X-ray.

Cushing's concept of a pituitary origin of the syndrome was based on clinical and postmortem studies of several patients.

It then gradually came to be realized that the tumor need not necessarily be bulky, but, quite to the contrary, striking clinical effects might be produced by minute, symptomatic predictable adenomas. So it is the degree of secretory activity of an adenomata, which may be out of all proportion to its dimensions, that evokes the recognizable symptom-complex in all hypersecretory states.

In this review, Cushing noted that the first pathological demonstration of a millet seed-sized pituitary adenoma, accompanied by slightly enlarged adrenal glands and associated with signs and symptoms of Cushing's disease, was reported in 1915 by a Dr. J. Anderson, who believed it to be a case of hypopituitarism with secondary adrenal hyperfunction. Two other cases showing similar clinical manifestations in association with small pituitary adenomata were then reported, one by Dr. Zondek in 1923 and the other by Dr. Parkes-Weber in 1926. The latter, however, stated that there could be no connection between the pituitary tumor and the clinical features.

Cushing's awareness of the physiology of pituitary secretion and of pituitary structure subsequently enabled his junior co-worker, Dr. Teel, to predict in 1931, ante mortem, the presence of a small basophil adenoma in a patient with the manifestations of Cushing's disease. The concept of a pituitary etiology dominated the thinking of the following decade (Table 1.2). However, questions arose concerning the postulated etiological role of the pituitary, since investigators of this period were unable to demonstrate elevated plasma ACTH levels associated with this condition. What was not then fully realized was that this inability was due, in part, to (1) the insensitivity of available bioassays for ACTH, (2) the failure to realize that even normal levels of ACTH were inappropriate in the face of elevated plasma cortisol levels, and (3) the failure to appreciate the absence of normal circadian variation of plasma ACTH levels. In contrast to the afternoon and evening decreases in such levels in normal individuals, plasma ACTH

**Table 1.2.** Postulated etiologies of Cushing's disease [a]

| | | |
|---|---|---|
| 1930s | Pituitary | Cushing-basophilic adenomata or hyperplasia |
| 1940s | Adrenal | Hyperresponsiveness to ACTH |
| | | Cortisol-induced Crooke's changes |
| | Hypothalamus | Lesions in paraventricular (PV), SO nuclei |
| | | Cases associated with increased intracranial pressure 2° to CNS tumor regressing following tumor removal |
| | | Evidence of increased intracranial pressure and cortical atrophy at postmortem or by PEG in cases of Cushing's disease |
| 1950s–1970s | Pituitary | Efficacy of pituitary irradiation |
| | | Efficacy of microadenomectomy |
| 1970s | Hypothalamus | Other associated neuroendocrine abnormalities |
| | | Sleep EEG abnormalities |
| | | Response to antiserotonergic, antidopaminergic agents |

[a] The third column cites basis for ascribing such etiology (see text).

in patients with Cushing's disease remains at the same level throughout the 24-h period, resulting in a greater amount of ACTH secreted per day, even though morning levels are "normal." This fact was subsequently highlighted by the observations by Nugent et al. (1960) that infusions of ACTH over several days at constant rates, in such small amounts that they did not reach detectable concentrations in blood, resulted in elevated arrhythmic plasma cortisol concentration. The presence of an 8%–20% incidence of pituitary tumors seen at autopsy in endocrinologically normal subjects also raised some questions as to the functional significance of adenomata found in patients with Cushing's disease, even though, as will be discussed later, the incidence of such adenomata was much higher among these patients than among normal subjects.

During the 1940s, two etiological theories were invoked. According to the first, the defect was at the adrenal level. Supporters of this theory cited the adrenal hyperresponsiveness to ACTH in this condition, as well as the presence of Crooke's hyaline changes in the anterior pituitary (seen under conditions of both exogenous and endogenous hypercortisolism), as evidence for a primary adrenal etiology, any pituitary changes being secondary. Other observations, however, suggested a central nervous system (CNS) etiology. Lesions in the paraventricular and supraoptic nuclei were noted at autopsy of patients with Cushing's disease (Heinbecker 1944). There were also reports of cases associated with increased intracranial pressure secondary to CNS tumors in which the symptoms of Cushing's disease regressed following tumor removal (although today ectopic ACTH production by such tumors should also be considered). Still other reports described evidence of increased intracranial pressure and cortical atrophy postmortem or by pneumoencephalography (PEG) in some cases of Cushing's disease.

From the 1950s to the present, it has once again been felt that the primary etiology lies within the pituitary gland. Supporters of this view point to the efficacy of pituitary irradiation in amelioration of this syndrome (although it should also be noted that the hypothalamus is more radiosensitive than the pituitary), and to the more recent reports of cure by microadenomectomy.

A hypothalamic etiology has also been considered, in view of the known regulation of ACTH release by a still unidentified hypothalamic corticotropin-releasing factor (CRF). This is suggested by studies of patients with Cushing's disease reporting (1) altered neuroendocrine parameters of several hormones in addition to ACTH, (2) disturbances in sleep EEG in states of clinical activity and in remission, (3) a therapeutic response of some patients to agents that effect CNS neurotransmitter concentrations or action, (4) the presence of basophil hyperplasia rather than adenomata in some patients, and (5) the recurrence of disease in some patients following microadenomectomy. The following chapters will consider the normal regulation of ACTH secretion, the physiological effects of ACTH and of corticosteroids, the evidence of hypersecretion of related peptides in this condition, and the clinical, pathological, and laboratory abnormalities associated with the various etiologies of Cushing's disease and syndrome, as well as current modalities of treatment.

Since its initial description, Cushing's disease has fascinated many investigators by providing a pathophysiological disturbance that requires an understanding of normal regulatory processes concerned with ACTH chemistry and secretion. This understanding, by illuminating many aspects of such regulatory processes, can lead to more effective modalities for control of the disease.

## References

Anderson J (1915) A case of polyglandular syndrome with adrenal hypernephroma and adenoma on the pituitary gland—both of small size. Glasgow Med J 83:178–192

Cushing H (1932) The basophil adenomas of the pituitary body and their clinical manifestations. Bull Johns Hopkins Hosp 1(3):137–195

Heinbecker P (1944) Pathogenesis of Cushing's syndrome. Medicine 23:225–247

Nugent CA, Eik-Nes K, Kent HS, Samuels LT Tyler FH (1960) A possible explanation for Cushing's syndrome associated with adrenal hyperplasia. J Clin Endocrinol 20:1259–1268

Parkes WF (1926) Cutaneous striae, purpura, high blood-pressure, amenorrhoea and obesity, of the type sometimes connected with cortical tumours of the adrenal glands, occurring in the absence of any such tumour—with some remarks on the morphogenetic and hormonic effects of the true hypernephromata of the adrenal cortex. Br J Dermatol 38:1–19

Teel HM (1931) Basophilic adenoma of the hypophysis with associated pluriglandular syndrome. Arch Neurol Psychiatr 26:593–599

Zondek H (1923) Die Krankheiten der endokrinen Drüsen. Springer, Berlin, p 287

*Chapter 2*

# Physiology of Regulation of ACTH Secretion

## A. Chemistry of ACTH

ACTH, as originally isolated from the pituitary gland and subsequently synthesized, is a single-chain polypeptide containing 39 amino acids, which stimulates the adrenal cortex in vertebrate animals and man. The N-terminal 24 amino acids are identical in all species studied. Minor species differences in amino acid composition occur in the 25–39 portion of the molecule. On a molar basis, the 1–24 amino acid sequence of the ACTH molecule possesses biological steroidogenic activity equivalent to that of the $ACTH^{1-39}$ molecule. There is a marked loss of steroidogenic potency with sequences smaller than $ACTH^{1-18}$. The duration of action is also diminished by deletion of COOH terminal sequences (Schwyzer 1964).

It has recently been demonstrated that $ACTH^{1-39}$ derives from a larger precursor molecule (31K ACTH/endorphin, pro-opiocortin) which also contains the sequence of $\beta$-lipotropin (Fig. 2.1.) (Mains et al. 1977; Roberts and Herbert 1977; Rubinstein et al. 1978; Roberts et al. 1978; Eipper and Mains 1978). The function of $\beta$-lipotropin is thus far unknown. There have been no studies on the physiological significance of its lipotropic activities.

The large precursor form of ACTH is a glycoprotein. It is currently believed that the initial translation product is a 28.5K nonglycosylated form which subsequently undergoes variable glycosylation, as indicated in Fig. 2.2. From this figure, it becomes apparent that each of the large glycosylated forms gives rise to an intermediate-size glycosylated ACTH form and to lipotropin. These intermediate forms of ACTH vary in size from 13–23K. The larger glycosylated forms (21–31K) have limited biological activity, which may be inherent in the molecule or may represent the biological activity of smaller forms generated in the course of extraction of the larger forms. The forms are subsequently processed to $ACTH^{1-39}$. The 13K glycosylated form is fully active as $ACTH^{1-39}$. It should be noted that the indicated molecular weights are only approximate, as they refer to mouse tumor ACTH; there is evidence of interspecies variation in the molecular size of the precursor molecules.

Both $ACTH^{1-39}$ and $\beta$-lipotropin can be processed further to other small peptides. Some of these are also biologically active, although not necessarily with regard to stimulation of the adrenal cortex (see below). In the anterior pituitary, $ACTH^{1-39}$ appears to be secreted without further processing (Lowry and Scott 1975); there is still some question as to the extent and circumstances under which $\beta$-lipotropin undergoes further processing to $\beta$-endorphin and to $\gamma$-LPH in this lobe (Scott and Lowry 1974; Guillemin et al. 1977; Liotta et al. 1978; Suda et al. 1978; Tanaka et al. 1978). The previous reports of β-MSH in pituitary extracts and in plasma are now realized to be secondary to an artifact occasioned by the extraction methodology employed for assay, β-MSH being generated therein by enzymatic cleavage from β-LPH (Scott and Lowry 1974).

In recent years, the demonstration of β-endorphin and related opioid peptides in the brain has occasioned much speculation regarding their role in pain perception and disease. Their derivation from a precursor molecule present in the brain, similar or identical to pro-opiocortin, is beyond the scope of this chapter (Krieger and Liotta 1979). The functional significance of circulating plasma β-endorphin and the stimuli that regulate it remain to be demonstrated (see below). Similarly, nothing is thus far known of the function of the portion of the precursor molecule present in addition to ACTH and LPH. As indicated in Fig. 2.1, a fragment (γ-MSH) is present, with marked homologies to other melanocyte-stimulating hormones in the molecule, and its presence in peripheral circulation has been demonstrated. It is possible that this portion of the molecule may also serve as a precursor to other unidentified peptides. High molecular weight material represents a very small, variable proportion of immunoreactive ACTH-like material in normal human plasma (Ratter et al. 1980).

In those species posessing an intermediate lobe, it is believed that $ACTH^{1-39}$ itself acts as a precursor molecule which is enzymatically cleaved to α-MSH (acetyl-$ACTH^{1-13}$ amide) and CLIP (corticotropin-like intermediate-lobe peptide) ($ACTH^{18-39}$) (Lowry and Scott 1975), while β-LPH is cleaved to γ-LPH (β-$LPH^{1-58}$), β-endorphin (β-$LPH^{61-91}$), and possibly β-MSH (β-$LPH^{41-58}$) (Lowry and Scott 1975; Crine et al. 1978). α-MSH and β-MSH have melanocyte-stimulating activity in lower vertebrate forms and in the human fetus. It has also been suggested that α-MSH may stimulate cortisol secretion (Glickman et al. 1979). The function of CLIP is unknown, though stimulation of insulin secretion has been suggested.

It is evident that any consideration of ACTH secretion regulation should consider the species involved, as well as possible regulatory alterations of other components of the precursor molecule. However, a complete understanding of this is not presently available.

## B. Histology

The concept of a prohormone for ACTH and LPH is also confirmed by histological studies. It has been shown that in the human, as well as other species, the prohormone "31K ACTH," ACTH, and β-lipotropin all occur within the same cell (Pelletier et al. 1977; Pelletier et al. 1979), and possibly within the same secretory granule. A specific cell type has been identified in rat pituitary, which is a stellate cell with a size and granule content that varies with corticosteroid level (Siperstein and Miller 1973). The size of this cell increases after adrenalectomy. A decreased number of granules is present 24 h after adrenalectomy in parallel with the known decrease in pituitary ACTH content at that time. A marked increase in cytoplasmic granulation is seen 1 week postadrenalectomy concomitant with the presence of in-

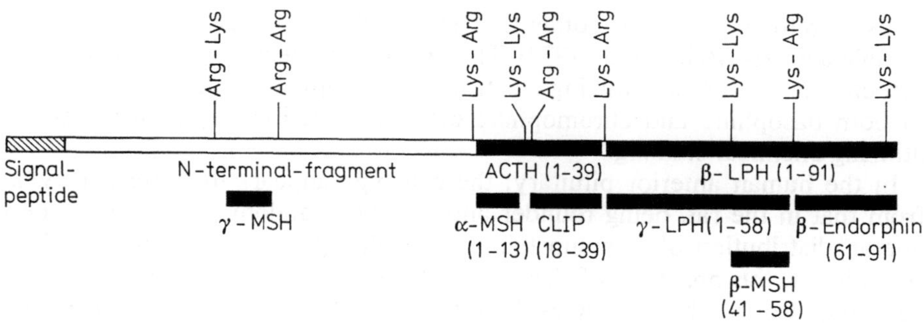


**Fig. 2.1.** Schematic representation of the bovine precursor molecule as proposed by Nakanishi et al. (1979). Following the signal peptide, there is an N-terminal fragment followed by $ACTH^{1-39}$, followed by the $\beta$-lipotropin$^{1-91}$ sequence. $\gamma$-MSH (melanocyte-stimulating hormone) refers to the sequence of amino acid residues −55 to −44 (amino acid residues N-terminal to the ACTH sequence are given minus designation) in the N-terminal fragment as determined from the cloned complementary DNA sequence of a mRNA molecule. $ACTH^{1-39}$ contains within it the sequences of $\alpha$-MSH and CLIP (corticotropin-like intermediate-lobe peptide). $\beta$-Lipotropin contains the sequences of $\gamma$-lipotropin, $\beta$-MSH, and $\beta$-endorphin. Note that all the indicated peptide fragments are flanked on both sides by a pair of basic amino acid residues that can potentially be proteolytically cleaved to yield the component peptides

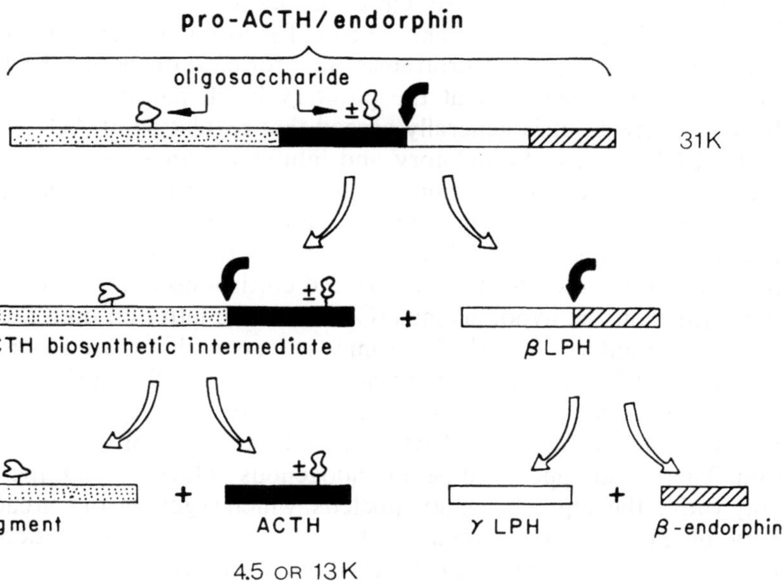


**Fig. 2.2.** Schemata of glycosylation ( , ) of the pro-ACTH/endorphin molecule: (±) indicates form may be either glycosylated or unglycosylated. (From R. Mains, personal com-

creased pituitary ACTH content. These cells are larger in female than in male animals (Baker et al. 1970). They have been demonstrated by immunocytochemical methods utilizing electron microscopy and appear to be similar to both basophilic and chromophilic cells, as described by earlier methods utilizing chemical staining.

In the human anterior pituitary, the cell type appears to differ somewhat from that in the rat, being rounder and having a random, rather than a peripheral, distribution of immunostaining granules (Halmi and Moriarty 1977). In addition, the presence of dense vesicles has been reported in the human corticolipotroph. These vesicles do not stain with anti-ACTH or anti-$\beta$-LPH, suggesting two subpopulations of secretory granules. The function of the unstained granules remains completely unknown (Pelletier et al. 1978). The human corticolipotroph has been shown to undergo Crooke's changes, in the presence of excess exogenous or endogenous corticosteroids, by electron microscopy. These changes represent massive accumulation of filaments, and have thus far been seen only in human pituitary. The nature of the basophils in pars nervosa of human beings is still unclear. An early study (Morris et al. 1956) indicated that these cells contained MSH but little or no bioactive ACTH, although they did stain with antibody against $ACTH^{17-39}$ (Phifer et al. 1974). There have been no studies to date utilizing immunocytochemistry with the aid of antibodies against the bioactive portions of ACTH and $\beta$-lipotropin.

## C. Physiology of ACTH Secretion

ACTH is secreted in response to diverse stimuli. The regulation of its basal release, stress-evoked release, circadian periodicity, and modulation by corticosteroid feedback is probably accomplished via different neuroanatomical pathways and different neurotransmitters for each of these aspects. Although there is local modulation at the pituitary level, particularly with regard to feedback effects, it is generally agreed that regulation of ACTH secretion is under CNS control. Stimulatory and inhibitory inputs originating in various areas of the CNS synapse on a thus far uncharacterized group of neurosecretory cells, modulating their release of a thus far uncharacterized corticotropin-releasing factor (CRF)[1], which acts to increase both pituitary synthesis and release of ACTH. ACTH and cortisol both have feedback actions, the former on the hypothalamus (CRF) and the latter on both the hypothalamus and pituitary ACTH. Superimposed upon this closed-loop circuit are environmental and other endogenous inputs affecting higher CNS centers (i.e., stress, fever, changes in blood pressure and volume) that apparently act upon the hypothalamic CRF cells independently of any feedback regulation. There also appears to be an endogenous "clock" within the CNS, probably within the suprachiasmatic nucleus, which regulates the circadian periodicity of the pituitary-adrenal system. In the following sections, some of these aspects of ACTH regulation will be discussed in greater detail.

1 Vale et al. (Science 213:1394, 1981) have very recently reported characterization of a 41-residue ovine hypothalamic peptides that stimulates secretion of corticotropin and β-endorphin.

## I. Corticotropin-Releasing Factor

The presence of material capable of releasing ACTH was first described by Saffran et al. (1955) and Guillemin and Rosenberg (1955) in material from both posterior pituitary and hypothalamic tissue. This material was characterized as a peptide by Guillemin et al. (1957). Subsequent studies have demonstrated material with corticotropin-releasing-like activity both within and outside the hypothalamus (Yasuda and Greer 1976; Krieger et al. 1977). Recent studies report that although the highest concentrations of CRF activity in the hypothalamus were found in the median eminence (Krieger et al. 1977), even higher concentrations were present in infundibular stalk and posterior pituitary (Yasuda et al. 1977). Since hypothalamic deafferentation is associated with an increase in hypothalamic CRF content the source of CRF may be within this area (Krieger et al. 1977), although this has been questioned by Makara et al. (1979).

Since its initial description, many attempts have been made to purify and identify CRF. It was originally proposed that corticotropin-releasing activity might be present in several diverse polypeptides related either to α-MSH or to vasopressin (Schally et al. 1960). Whether vasopressin is CRF, a material with some CRF-like activity, or a cofactor of CRF is still a matter of controversy (Gillies and Lowry 1976; Krieger and Zimmerman 1977; Zimmerman et al. 1977). In vitro studies have reported contradictory results. Hypothalamic extracts from Brattleboro rats, animals lacking vasopressin, still have CRF-like activity. Immunocytochemical studies have provided evidence that, in addition to the classical pathway containing vasopressin arising from the supraoptic and paraventricular nuclei to the posterior pituitary, another pathway arises from the same nuclei and terminates in the median eminence in contact with the portal vascular system. This would permit transfer of centrally synthesized vasopressin to the anterior pituitary, in addition to any possible direct transfer of stored hormone from the posterior pituitary.

Preliminary reports indicated that CRF was a substance of molecular weight varying from 1200–1500 daltons and that it was peptide in nature. A large molecular weight form has also been described in hypophyseal stalk (Yasuda et al. 1978). In addition, there have been reports of CRF-like material present in extracranial tissue (Brodish 1977) and plasma (Hagen et al. 1977). Thus far, there is no information as to whether these are physicochemically or structurally identical to CRF found in hypothalamus and posterior pituitary. The only currently available method for measurement of CRF is by determination of its ACTH-releasing activity. This type of bioassay may measure a variety of substances with ACTH-releasing activity, so it is uncertain that all the described forms are chemically similar.

Very recently, Vale et al. (1981) have described isolation from ovine hypothalami of a 41-residue amidated peptide which is highly active in stimulating the secretion of ACTH and β-endorphin in vitro from anterior pituitary cell cultures. The relation of these peptides to those partially purified molecules described by others cannot be determined without direct chemical and biological comparison. Of great interest is the observation of an approximately 50% homology of this CRF with amino acids present in sauvagine, a 40-residue peptide isolated from frog skin.

There is disagreement regarding the effect of hormonal manipulation on CRF content. Krieger et al. (1977) report that dexamethasone treatment and hypophysectomy increase hypothalamic CRF content, but no such effect has been found by Yasuda and Greer (1976).

CRF is believed to increase both synthesis and release of ACTH. The effect on the latter is extremely rapid (Mulder and Smelik 1977). This is compatible with the findings that electrical (Grizzle et al. 1974) or chemical (Krieger and Krieger 1970b) stimulation of the hypothalamus in vivo results in increased plasma ACTH concentrations within 1 min.

It has been reported that the effect of CRF on release of ACTH by the anterior pituitary is blocked in vitro by substance P (Jones et al. 1978b), somatostatin (Voigt et al., 1976), melanocyte hormone-inhibiting factor (Voigt et al. 1976), prostaglandins, and corticosteroids. In vivo studies with melanocyte hormone-inhibiting factor have been contradictory (Donnadieu et al. 1976). It remains to be seen whether additional in vivo studies confirm any other in vitro effects and whether these will be clinically relevant. There is one report of decreased plasma ACTH concentrations in humans following somatostatin administration (Tyrrell 1975).

Finally, a direct stimulatory effect of norepinephrine on ACTH release in dispersed pituitary cells has been demonstrated (Vale and Rivier 1977). The response to norepinephrine and other $\alpha$-adrenergic agonists can be distinguished from that seen with hypothalamic extract. The significance of these observations is unknown. At present, therefore, there is evidence of several kinds of CRF-like materials: those of neural origin; those of extraneural origin; vasopressin; and perhaps a neurotransmitter, such as norepinephrine.

## II. Neurotransmitter Regulation of ACTH Release

A considerable body of information exists concerning the role of neurotransmitters believed to regulate CRF release, although there are inconsistencies in the reported data. Some of these inconsistencies appear related to performance of studies in different species, at different times of day, and studies in anesthetized or stressed animals (both of the latter variables may influence the effect of any postulated neurotransmitter being tested). It has been demonstrated (Krieger and Krieger 1970a, b) that cholinergic drugs, norepinephrine, $\gamma$-aminobutyric acid (GABA), and serotonin can stimulate ACTH release, presumably CRF mediated, when implanted in different areas of the CNS. These studies have also indicated that a given transmitter can activate CRF release only in certain areas, since a given area may respond to one neurotransmitter and not to another. The median eminence was the only area where all neurotransmitters tested were effective. This area may serve as a common final pathway in the synaptic regulation of CRF release. In vitro studies by Jones et al. (1978a) postulated a model in which the CRF-containing cell is stimulated via a cholinergic input. The cholinergic cell itself may be presynaptically activated by serotonergic inputs, explaining the

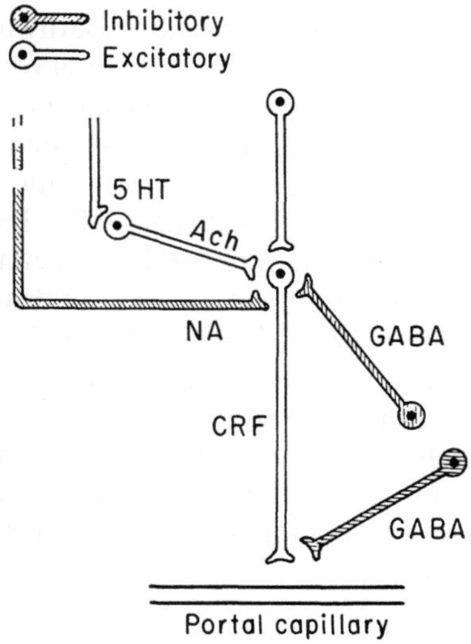


**Fig. 2.3.** Suggested model for the control of CRF from the hypothalamus. The model shows the CRF neuron with its axon terminating at a portal capillary; a serotonin *(5-HT)* pathway that releases CRF after excitation of a cholinergic interneuron; and the final common pathway to CRF release, which is cholinergic. Two cholinergic neurons are shown. One is the interneuron placed between the 5-HT pathway and the CRF cell (for control of the circadian rhythm?), the other cholinergic neuron does not have a 5-HT synapse and may control the stress-induced release of CRF. A noradrenergic pathway *(NA)*, which is inhibitory to CRF secretion, and a GABA inhibitory neuron are also shown. This could be either a pre- or postsynaptic input. From Jones and Hillhouse (1977a) with permission

stimulatory role noted for serotonin. In this system, norepinephrine had no direct stimulatory effect on CRF release, but blocked acetylcholine-stimulated release. An inhibitory GABA interneuron was also postulated, which was activated by stimulation of the CRF-producing neuron, thus providing a method for local feedback (Fig. 2.3). It has also become apparent that a given transmitter can affect the various parameters of ACTH release differentially. Cholinergic and serotonergic mechanisms appear to be involved in the circadian release of ACTH, whereas stress responses may have cholinergic and adrenergic or dopaminergic components, the latter of which may be inhibitory (Krieger et al. 1968; Krieger and Rizzo 1969; Ganong 1977). It should be realized that excitation of ACTH release can occur either by increasing excitatory impulses, decreasing inhibitory impulses, or as a result of a combination of these.

## III. Neuroanatomical Pathways Involved in ACTH Release

There are multiple inputs to the hypothalamus from the median forebrain bundle, limbic system areas, and supraoptic and paraventricular areas. Terminals from these areas may make contact with the CRF-releasing cell by axoaxonic or axodendritic, as well as by classical postsynaptic junctions. Again, it is believed that different aspects of CRF-mediated ACTH release are regulated by different neuroanatomic pathways, each of these possibly using different transmitters among those described above. It is clear that regulation of circadian periodicity of the pituitary-adrenal cortical system is effected via pathways entering from the anterior region of the hypothalamus (see below). Stress activation of CRF-ACTH release is believed to be mediated via pathways entering the hypothalamus posteriorly from the midbrain and pons (Slusher 1964). Although a corticotropin-release inhibitory factor has not been identified, there is neuroanatomical evidence for pathways that inhibit CRF release. These arise from the limbic system, particularly the hippocampal area (Raisman 1970).

In addition to neural pathways believed to effect CRF release, there is evidence of sympathetic nervous innervation of the anterior pituitary arising from the superior cervical ganglion via blood vessels to the pituitary. The functional significance of such innervation is still unknown, as is the significance of both serotonin and norepinephrine within the anterior pituitary (Hyyppa and Wurtman 1973; Piezzi et al. 1970). This latter finding is in keeping with the proposed characterization of pituitary cells as being part of the amine-precursor uptake and decarboxylation (APUD) series (Pearse and Takor 1976). This series includes groups of cells derived from neuroectoderm, and includes, in addition to the pituitary, thyroid C cells, adrenal medullary cells, pancreatic, stomach, intestinal, and specialized pulmonary cells. Such cells have two distinctive features; production of peptide hormones and the capability for APUD. The physiological significance of such an association of monoamines and peptides within the same APUD cell is unclear.

## IV. Feedback Regulation of ACTH

Both increases and decreases in corticosteroid concentrations affect pituitary ACTH secretion and release. The effects of acute and chronic alterations of such concentrations may differ (see below). There has been considerable dispute as to whether the site of positive steroid feedback (i.e., increased corticosteroid concentrations) lies within the pituitary or within the CNS.

Concerning the effect of "acute" corticosteroid elevation on feedback regulation of ACTH, corticosteroids, as shown by in vitro studies, can directly inhibit both pituitary ACTH synthesis and release, the former by depressing the intracellular level of the mRNA coding for the ACTH precursor (Nakanishi et al. 1977). Corticosteroids also interfere with CRF-induced release of ACTH from the pituitary. This effect requires pituitary pretreatment by dexamethasone before exposure to CRF. This blocking effect of dexamethasone can be prevented by pretreatment with actinomycin-D, an inhibitor of DNA-dependent RNA synthesis (Arimura et al. 1969). There is also evidence for feedback at the hypothalamic level. Earlier studies on hypothalamic implantation (Chowers et al. 1963; Zimmerman and Critchlow 1969a) were criticized for assuming that such intracerebrally injected hydrocortisone was really diffusing into the pituitary and having a local site of action. However, a direct effect of corticosteroids on in vitro hypothalamic release of CRF has been reported (Jones et al. 1977b). It has also been shown that corticosteroids are taken up and concentrated in the hypothalamus as well as in limbic system areas, with greater uptake in the latter.

Consideration of feedback becomes more complicated with the recognition that two types of feedback exist at both the pituitary and hypothalamic levels (Jones et al. 1977b): a rapid, rate-sensitive feedback (Dallman and Yates 1969) and a delayed, level-sensitive feedback (Smelik 1963; Yates and Maran 1974; Fehm et al. 1979). The delayed feedback mechanism may be accomplished by inhibition of ACTH synthesis via cortisol binding to intracytosol receptors with nuclear transfer and action on the genome, as well as by an additional effect on ACTH release. The fast feedback mechanism may involve some type of membrane effect, as yet uncharacterized. That the two feedback mechanisms have different loci of action is also supported by the observation that these mechanisms are affected in different ways by several steroids (Jones et al. 1974). In the pituitary, in addition to specific cytosol corticosteroid receptors, transcortin-like material is present within the pituitary cell membrane (DeKloet et al. 1977; Maclusky et al. 1977). Since various steroids have differential binding affinities for transcortin and for cytosol receptors, this may, in part, explain some of their differential effects. In brain, transcortin-like material is absent. However, the existence therein of more than one population of receptor sites, differing in steroid specificity and regional distribution, has been inferred by competition experiments utilizing dexamethasone and corticosterone (McEwen 1977).

In addition to affecting basal secretion, administration of corticosteroids will suppress the subsequent circadian peak of plasma corticosteroid concentrations (Zimmerman and Critchlow 1969b; Krieger et al. 1971). Such suppression is most effective when the exogenous glucocorticoid is administered several hours prior to the time of the expected circadian peak. Acute elevation of plasma corticosteroid concentrations by exogenous steroid administration will also suppress stress-induced release of ACTH. Such studies have demonstrated that the magnitude of this effect is a function of the time of pretreatment with the synthetic steroid, and also varies with the stress employed (Takebe et al. 1968; Sirett and Gibbs 1969; Takebe et al. 1971). The physiological implications of these observations are somewhat unclear. The studies cited measure the effect of administration of an exogenous corticosteroid prior to stress on the subsequent corticosteroid response to the stress. However, in clinical situations one is more concerned with the effect of the physiological increase in corticosteroid concentrations produced by stress on the subsequent functioning of the CNS-pituitary-adrenal system. It has been shown in the experimental animal that elevation of plasma corticosteroid concentrations by stress does not alter the ACTH release occasioned by a subsequent stress (Dallman and Jones 1973).

Concerning the effect of chronic elevation of corticosteroid levels, considerable individual variation may be noted in the rate of recovery of pituitary-adrenal function, partly dependent on the dose and duration of preceding corticosteroid administration. Serial measurements following discontinuation of long-term corticosteroid treatment or removal of an adrenal adenoma show that decreased plasma ACTH and corticosteroid concentrations are present initially, secondary to decreased pituitary synthesis and release of ACTH. There is a subsequent increase to "supernormal" plasma ACTH concentrations within 2–5 months (still accompanied by decreased plasma corticosteroid concentrations because of decreased adrenal responsiveness to ACTH). Finally, within a 4–9-month period, normal plasma ACTH and corticosteroid concentrations are achieved (Graber et al. 1965). With resumption of normal adrenal responsiveness to ACTH, there is concomitant return of normal responsiveness to hypoglycemia and to vasopressin (Pitressin). Resumption of circadian periodicity appears to take somewhat longer (Krieger and Gewirtz 1974b).

As to the effect of decreased corticosterone concentration, adrenalectomy in the rat is associated with a rapid rise in plasma ACTH concentrations within 2.5 min, followed by a gradual decline; a plateau is reached between 2–12 h subsequently and continues until 4 days following adrenalectomy, after which time persistently elevated levels are seen (Dallman et al. 1972; Buckingham and Hodges 1974). The decrease in plasma ACTH concentrations is accompanied by a concomitant decrease in those of pituitary ACTH, which then rises to greater than normal concentrations parallel with those of plasma ACTH. It should be noted that during the plateau phase, plasma ACTH concentrations in adrenalectomized animals remain higher than those seen in sham-adrenalectomized animals, and are not suppressible to the same extent as in normal subjects (Buckingham and Hodges 1974; Krieger and Gewirtz 1974a). Studies in human subjects have been performed only in Addisonian patients in whom corticosteroid replacement therapy has been briefly discontinued. Such subjects display markedly elevated plasma ACTH concentrations when sampled 12 h after receiving their last dose of medication. Perhaps more similar to studies on adrenalectomized animals are those in which human subjects have been given large oral doses of metyrapone, which induces elevated plasma ACTH levels within 1 h of drug administration (Hawano et al. 1972).

### V. Circadian Periodicity

It is believed that the circadian periodicity of the CNS-pituitary-adrenal system is an endogenous one. Its phase, however, can be regulated by external influences. Both light-dark and sleep-wake transitions have been implicated as phase regulators, with peak hormone concentrations seen just prior to, or at the time of awakening. A period of 7–9 days is required for phase reversal of this periodicity to occur following reversal of light-dark, sleep-wake conditions.

Circadian periodicity is evident at all levels of the CNS-pituitary-adrenal axis (Krieger 1977) (Fig. 2.4). A circadian periodicity of metabolic pattern and corticosteroid secretion in cultured hamster adrenal glands has been reported (Andrews and Folk 1964), although this has not been confirmed in studies utilizing monolayer cultures from adrenal cortical cells (O'Hare and Hornsby 1974). A circadian variation in adrenal responsiveness to ACTH has been demonstrated in animal studies (Dallman 1976), but not in human studies (Nugent et al. 1960; Ungar and Halberg 1962). Circadian variation in plasma corticosteroid concentrations has also been reported in hypophysectomized fish (Srivasian and Meier 1972) and rats (Meier 1976). However, in addition to whatever evidence exists for periodicity at the adrenal level, there is evidence in both adrenalectomized animals and humans (Cheifetz et al. 1968; Krieger and Gewirtz 1974a) of a circadian periodicity in plasma ACTH levels (Fig. 2.5). This would imply a regulatory mechanism at the pituitary level superimposed upon any inherent adrenal rhythm. This observation also indicates that the pattern of plasma ACTH concentrations is not generated by corticosteroid feedback regulation, although the lack of such feedback results in higher ACTH concentrations at any given point in the circadian cycle.

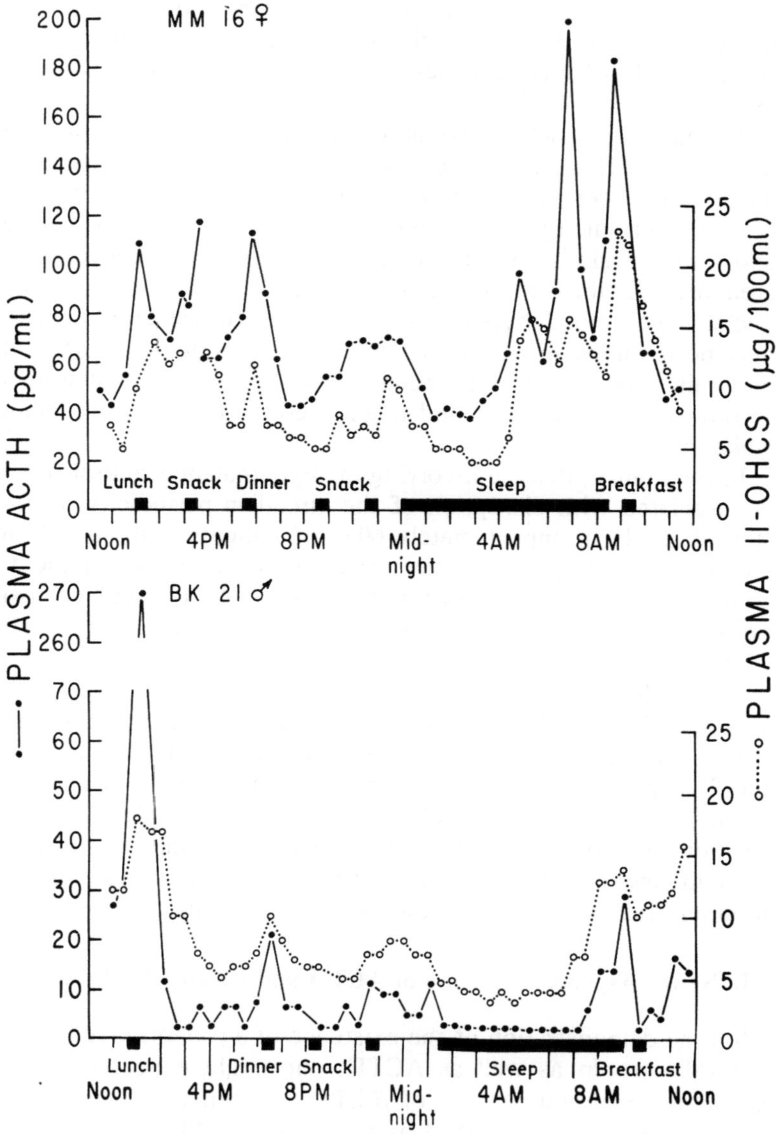


**Fig. 2.4.** Circadian periodicity of plasma 11-OHCS and plasma ACTH levels over a 24-h period as determined by half-hourly samples. Mealtimes and sleep as indicated. From Krieger et al. (1971) with permission

There is also a circadian periodicity of corticotropin-releasing activity in rat hypothalamus (Hiroshige and Sato 1970), which persists in hypophysectomized animals (Takebe 1972). Such periodicity becomes evident at the same age (i.e., the prepubertal period) as the appearance of circadian periodicity of plasma corticosteroid levels. Serotonergic and cholinergic mediation of circadian corticosteroid periodicity has been documented in both human and animal studies (Krieger and Krieger 1967a, b; Chihara et al. 1976; Ferrari et al. 1977). A regional circadian periodicity of these neurotransmitters within the CNS has been described (Hanin et al. 1970; Simon and George 1975).

Although the exact neuroanatomical pathways involved in circadian periodicity of ACTH release have not been fully delineated, the suprachiasmatic nucleus has been implicated as the major neural area involved in regulation of such periodicity (Moore and Eichler 1972). There is dense cholinergic and serotonergic innervation of this area. Two of the afferent inputs to this area are via the retinohypothalamic tracts and from the midbrain raphe nuclei. The retinal hypothalamic pathway to the suprachiasmatic nucleus may be involved in light-dark regulation of periodicity, while that from the midbrain raphe nuclei has been implicated in the regulation of sleep via serotonergic mechanisms and might mediate the phase regulation by sleep-wake transition.

In the human, disease involving the hypothalamus and/or the limbic system is associated with disruption of the circadian periodicity of plasma corticosteroid levels in approximately 60% of patients with such lesions (Krieger and Krieger 1966). The pattern seen in some of these patients consists of completely random episodic variations of ACTH and cortisol concentrations, reminiscent of the pattern observed in patients with Cushing's disease (Krieger et al. 1971).

When the circadian periodicity of plasma corticosteroid concentrations was initially described, it was depicted as a curve where attainment of peak levels was followed by a smooth progressive fall during the remainder of the 24-h period. It is now apparent that there is evidence of episodic secretion superimposed on such a pattern (Krieger et al. 1971) (Fig. 2.4). Similar episodic secretion of ACTH is also seen in adrenalectomized subjects (Krieger and Gewirtz 1974a). Because of technical difficulties, it is not yet possible to determine whether CRF concentrations also vary episodically.

## VI. Newer Aspects of Release of ACTH and Related Peptides

With the demonstration of the existence of a prohormone for ACTH containing $\beta$-lipotropin as well as ACTH, one might expect concurrent secretion of $\beta$-lipotropin and perhaps of $\beta$-LPH fragments with ACTH, in response to factors previously described as regulating ACTH release. In human studies to date, plasma $\beta$-lipotropin levels appear to exhibit parallel responses to those of ACTH with regard to circadian periodicity, response to corticosteroid administration, and responses to insulin-induced hypoglycemia and vasopressin. $\beta$-LPH appears to be secreted in amounts equimolar to those of ACTH, which would be in keeping with the structure of the prohormone molecule. Plasma endorphin concentrations, however, are barely detectable in many human subjects. They have been reported to increase in response to metyrapone administration (Krieger 1978), as well as to insulin-induced hypoglycemia (Imura et al. 1979). It remains to be seen whether these and other stresses and alterations in steroid concentrations can alter the processing either of the prohormone or of its constituents, permitting generation under such condi-

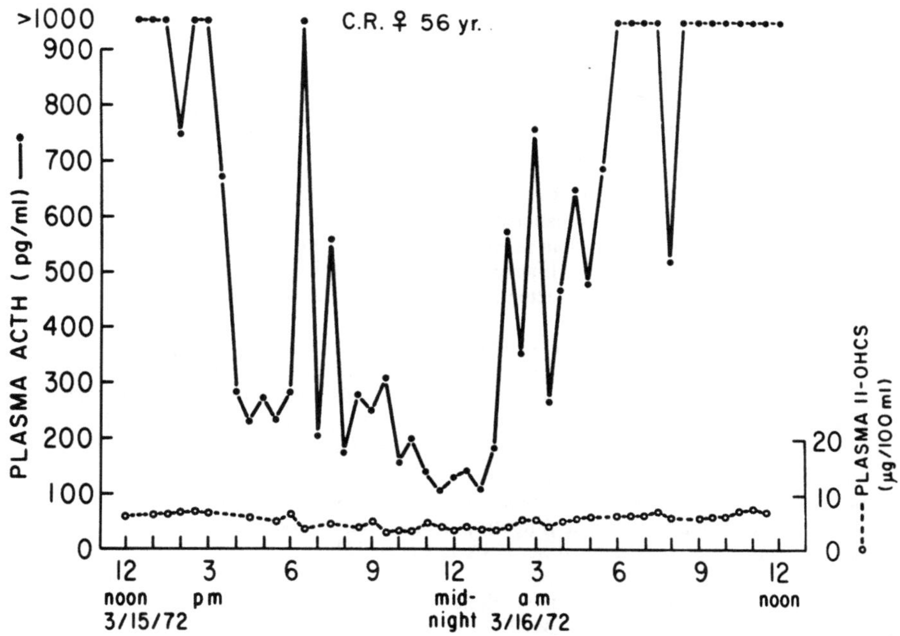


**Fig. 2.5.** Plasma ACTH and cortisol levels as determined by half-hourly sampling in a patient with Addison's disease (last dose of cortisone acetate 16h prior to sampling). From Krieger and Gewirtz (1974b) with permission

tions of circulating peptide fragments that are not detectable in the basal state. The foregoing observations apply to anterior pituitary secretion of these peptides since, as previously noted, the adult human does not have a discrete intermediate lobe, although a variable number of intermediate-lobe-like cells have been described as invading the posterior lobe (Morris et al. 1956).

To date, studies of the intermediate lobe indicate that it does not secrete functionally significant amounts of ACTH in response to stress, and that its content of immunoreactive and bioreactive ACTH is not affected by adrenalectomy or by dexamethasone administration (Moriarty and Moriarty 1975). It does secrete $\alpha$-MSH in response to stress. The reported rise in plasma $\beta$-endorphin concentrations seen in stressed animals may well represent, in large part, intermediate lobe secretion (Guillemin et al. 1977). Serotonin is believed to directly stimulate intermediate lobe secretion, while dopamine (DA) is inhibitory. There is some disagreement as to whether or not median eminence extract effects release of ACTH from this lobe.

In view of the rapid expansion of studies in this field, it is evident that in the future it will be necessary to reevaluate mechanisms governing the secretion of the extended family of ACTH-like peptides.

## References


Andrews RF, Folk GE Jr (1964) Circadian metabolic patterns in cultured hamster glands. J Comp Biochem Physiol 2:393–409

Arimura A, Bowers CY, Schally AV, Saito M, Miller MC (1969) Effect of corticotrophin-releasing factor, dexamethasone and actinomycin-D on the release of ACTH from rat pituitaries in vivo and in vitro. Endocrinology 85:300–311

Baker BL, Pek S, Midgley AR Jr, Gersten BE (1970) Identification of the corticotropin cell in rat hypophyses with peroxidase-labeled antibody. Anat Rec 166:557–568

Brodish A (1977) Tissue corticotropin-releasing factors. Fed Proc 36:2088–2093

Buckingham JC, Hodges JR (1974) Interrelationships of pituitary and plasma corticotrophin and plasma corticosterone in adrenalectomized and stressed, adrenalectomized rats. J Endocrinol 63:213–111

Cheifetz P, Gaffud N, Dingman JF (1968) Effects of bilateral adrenalectomy and continuous light on the circadian rhythms of corticotropin in female rats. Endocrinology 82:1117–1124

Chihara K, Kato Y, Maeda K, Matsukura S, Imura H (1976) Suppression by cyproheptadine of human growth hormone and cortisol secretion during sleep. J Clin Invest 57:1393–1402

Chowers I, Feldman S, Davidson JM (1963) Effects of intrahypothalamic crystalline steroids on acute ACTH secretion. Am J Physiol 205:671–673

Crine P, Gianoulakis C, Seidah NG, Gossard F, Pezalla PD, Lis M, Chretien M (1978) Biosynthesis of $\beta$-endorphin from $\beta$-lipotropin and a larger molecular weight precursor in rat pars intermedia. Proc Natl Acad Sci USA 75:4719–4723

Cushing H (1932) The basophil adenomas of the pituitary body and their clinical manifestations (pituitary basophilism). Bull Johns Hopkins Hosp 50:137–195

Dallman MF, Engeland WC, Shinsako J (1976) Circadian changes in adrenocortical response to ACTH. Prog 58th Meeting Endocrine Soc, p 58

Dallman MF, Jones MT (1973) Corticosteroid feedback control of ACTH secretion: Effect of stress-induced corticosterone secretion on subsequent stress responses in the rat. Endocrinology 92:1367–1375

Dallman MF, Jones MT, Vernikos-Danellis J (1972) Corticosteroid feedback control of ACTH secretion: Rapid effects of bilateral adrenalectomy on plasma ACTH in the rat. Endocrinology 91:961–968

Dallman MF, Yates FE (1969) Dynamic asymmetries in the corticosteroid feedback path and distribution-metabolism-binding elements of the adrenocortical system. Ann NY Acad Sci 156:696–721

DeKloet ER, Burbach P, Mulder GH (1977) Localization and role of transcortin-like molecules in the anterior pituitary. Mol Cell Endocrinol 7:261–273

Donnadieu M, Laurent MF, Luton JP, Bricaire H, Gerards F, Binoux M (1976) Synthetic MIF has no effect on $\beta$-MSH and ACTH hypersecretion in Nelson's syndrome. J Clin Endocrinol Metab 42:1145–1148

Eipper BA, Mains RE (1978) Analysis of the common precursor to corticotropin and endorphin. J Biol Chem 253:5732–5744

Fehm HL, Voigt KH, Kummer G, Lang R, Pfeiffer EF (1979) Differential and integral corticosteroid feedback effects on ACTH secretion in hypoadrenocorticism. J Clin Invest 63: 247–253

Ferrari E, Bosselo PA, Vailati A, Martinelli I, Rea A, Nosari I (1977) Variations circadiennes des effets d'une substance vagolytique sur le système ACTH-secrétant chez l'homme. Ann Endocrinol (Paris) 38:203–213

Ganong WF (1977) Neurotransmitters involved in ACTH secretion: Catecholamines. In: Krieger DT, Ganong WF (eds) ACTH and related peptides: Structure, regulation, and action. New York Academy of Sciences, New York, pp 509–517

Gillies G, Lowry P (1976) Investigation of CRF using the perfused anterior rat pituitary cell column. Proc. Vth Intl Congr Endocrinol 123

Glickman JA, Carson GD, Challis JRG (1979) Differential effects of synthetic adrenocorticotropin 1–24 and $\alpha$-melanocyte-stimulating hormone on adrenal function in human and sheep fetuses. Endocrinology 104:40–44

Graber AL, Ney RL, Nicholson WE (1965) Natural history of pituitary-adrenal recovery following long-term suppression with corticosteroids. J Clin Endocrinol 25:11–16

Grizzle WE, Dallman MF, Schramm LP (1974) Inhibitory and facilitatory hypothalamic areas mediating ACTH release in the cat. Endocrinology 95:1450–1461
Guillemin R, Hearn WR, Cheek WR, Housholder DE (1957) Control of corticotropin release: Further studies with in vitro methods. Endocrinology 60:488–506
Guillemin R, Rosenberg B (1955) Humoral hypothalamic control of anterior pituitary: A study with combined tissue cultures. Endocrinology 57:599–607
Guillemin R, Vargo T, Rossier J, Minnick S, Ling N, Rivier C, Vale W, Bloom F (1977) β-Endorphin and adrenocorticotropin are secreted concomitantly by the pituitary gland. Science 197:1367–1369
Hagen TC, Garthwaite TL, Martinson DR (1977) Circulating corticotropin-releasing factor-like activity in man. Proc Soc Exp Biol Med 156:518–522
Halmi NS, Moriarty GC (1977) The cells of origin of ACTH in man. In: Krieger DT, Ganong WF (eds) ACTH and related peptides. Ann NY Acad Sci 297:167–182
Hanin I, Massarelli R, Costa E (1970) Acetylcholine concentrations in rat brain: Diurnal oscillation. Science 170:341–342
Hawano S, Saito T, Shizume K (1972) Simultaneous determinations of plasma ACTH and GH levels after oral metyrapone. Endocrinol Jpn 19:477–481
Hiroshige T, Sato T (1970) Postnatal development of circadian rhythm of corticotropin-releasing activity in the rat hypothalamus. Endocrinol Jpn 17:106
Hyyppa M, Wurtman RJ (1973) Biogenic amines in the pituitary gland: What is their origin and function? Pituitary indolamines. Prog Brain Res 39:211–215
Imura H, Nakai Y, Nakao K, Jingami H (1979) Concomitant increase of plasma β-endorphin and ACTH levels in response to insulin-induced hypoglycemia in human subjects. Prog Endocrine Soc, 61st Meeting (Abstract)
Jones MT, Gillham B, Mahmoud S (1978a) Hypothalamus and ACTH secretion. In: James VHT, Serio M, Guisti G, Martini L (eds) The endocrine function of the human adrenal cortex. Academic Press, New York, pp 55–58
Jones MT, Guillemin R, Holmes MC, Hodges JR, Buckingham JC (1978b) Influence of substance P on hypothalamo-pituitary-adrenocortical activity in the rat. J Endocrinol 76:183–184
Jones MT, Hillhouse EW (1977a) Neurotransmitter regulation of corticotropin-releasing factor in vitro. In: Krieger DT, Ganong WF (eds) ACTH and related peptides: Structure, regulation and action. NY Acad Sci 297:536–560
Jones MT, Hillhouse EW, Burden JL (1977b) Dynamics and mechanics of corticosteroid feedback at the hypothalamus and anterior pituitary gland. J Endocrinol 73:405–417
Jones MT, Tiptaft EM, Brush FR, Fergusson DAN, Neame, RLB (1974) Evidence for dual corticosteroid-receptor mechanisms in the feedback control of adrenocorticotropin secretion. J Endocrinol 60:223–233
Krieger DT (1977) Regulation of circadian periodicity of plasma ACTH levels. In: Krieger DT, Ganong WF (eds) ACTH and related peptides: Structure, regulation and action. New York Academy of Sciences, New York, vol 297, pp 561–567
Krieger DT (1978) Plasma lipotropin and endorphin in the human. In: Graf L, Palkovits M, Ronai AZ (eds) Endorphins '78. Akademiai Kiado, Budapest, pp 275–294
Krieger DT, Allen W, Rizzo F, Krieger HP (1971) Characterization of the normal temporal pattern of plasma corticosteroid levels. J Clin Endocrinol Metab 32:266–284
Krieger DT, Gewirtz GP (1974a) Recovery of hypothalamic-pituitary-adrenal function, growth hormone responsiveness and sleep EEG pattern in a patient following removal of an adrenal cortical adenoma. J Clin Endocrinol Metab 38:1075–1082
Krieger DT, Gewirtz GP (1974b) The nature of the circadian periodicity and suppressibility of immunoreactive ACTH levels in Addison's disease. J Clin Endocrinol Metab 39:46–52
Krieger DT, Krieger HP (1967b) The effect of short-term administration of CNS-acting drugs on the circadian variation of the plasma 17-OHCS in normal subjects. Neuroendocrinology 2:232–246
Krieger DT, Krieger HP (1967a) Circadian pattern of plasma 17-hydroxycorticosteroids: Alteration by anticholinergic agents. Science 155:1421–1422
Krieger DT, Krieger HP (1966) The circadian variation of the plasma 17-OHCS in the central nervous system disease. J Clin Endocrinol 26:939–941
Krieger DT, Krieger HP (1970a) Effect of dexamethasone on pituitary-adrenal activation following intrahypothalamic implantation of neurotransmitters. Endocrinology 87:179–182

Krieger DT, Liotta AS (1979) Pituitary hormones in brain: Where, how, and why. Science 205: 366–205
Krieger DT, Liotta A, Brownstein MJ (1977) Corticotropin-releasing factor distribution in normal and Brattleboro rat brain, and effect of deafferentation hypophysectomy and steroid treatment in normal animals. Endocrinology 100:227–237
Krieger DT, Rizzo F (1969) Serotonin mediation of circadian periodicity of plasma 17-hydroxycorticosteroids. Am J Physiol 217:1703–1707
Krieger DT, Silverberg AI, Rizzo F, Krieger HP (1968) Abolition of circadian periodicity of plasma 17-OHCS levels in the cat. Am J Physiol 215:959–967
Krieger DT, Zimmermann EA (1977) The nature of CRF and its relationship to vasopressin. In: Martini L, Besser GM (eds) Clinical neuroendocrinology. Academic Press, New York, pp 363–391
Krieger HP, Krieger DT (1970b) Chemical stimulation of the brain: Effect on adrenal corticoid release. Am J Physiol 218:1632–1641
Liotta AS, Suda T, Krieger DT (1978) $\beta$-lipotropin is the major opioid-like peptide of human pituitary and rat pars distalis: Lack of significant $\beta$-endorphin. Proc Natl Acad Sci (USA 75:2950–2954
Lowry PJ, Scott AP (1975) The evolution of vertebrate corticotropin and melanocyte-stimulating hormone. Gen Comp Endocrinol 26:16–23
Maclusky NJ, Turner BB, McEwen BS (1977) Corticosteroid binding in rat brain and pituitary cytosols: Resolution of multiple binding components by polyacrylamide gel-based isoelectric focusing. Brain Res 130:564–571
Mains RE, Eipper BA, Ling N (1977) Common precursor to corticotropins and endorphins. Proc Natl Acad Sci USA 74:3014–3018
Makara GB, Stark E, Rappay G, Karteszi M, Palkovits M (1979) Changes in corticotropin releasing factor of the stalk median eminence in rats with various cuts around the medial basal hypothalamus. J Endocrinol 83:165–173
McEwen BS (1977) Adrenal steroid feedback on neuroendocrine tissues. In: Krieger DT, Ganong WF (eds) ACTH and related peptides: Structure, regulation and action. NY Acad Sci 297:568–579
Meier AH (1976) Daily variations in concentration of plasma corticosteroid in hypophysectomized rats. Endocrinology 98:1475–1479
Moore RY, Eichler VB (1972) Loss of a circadian adrenal corticosterone rhythm following suprachiasmatic lesions in the rat. Brain Res 42:201–206
Moriarty M, Moriarty GC (1975) Bioactive and immunoreactive ACTH in the rat pituitary. Endocrinology 96:1419–1425
Morris CJOR, Russell DS, Landgrebe FW, Mitchell GM (1956) The melanophore-expanding and corticotrophic activity of human pituitary tissue. J Endocrinol 14:263–267
Mulder GH, Smelik PG (1977) A superfusion system technique for the study of the sites of action of glucocorticoids in the rat hypothalamus-pituitary-adrenal system in vitro. I. Pituitary cell superfusion. Endocrinology 100:1143–1152
Nakanishi S, Inoue A, Kita T, Nakamura M, Chang ACY, Cohen SN, Numa S (1979) Nucleotide sequence of cloned cDNA for bovine corticotropin-$\beta$-lipotropin precursor. Nature 278: 423–427
Nakanishi S, Kita T, Taii S, Imura H, Numa S (1977) Glucocorticoid effect on the level of corticotropic messenger RNA activity in rat pituitary. Proc Natl Acad Sci USA 74:3283–3286
Nugent CA, Eik-Nes K, Kent HS, Samuels LT, Tyler FH (1960) A possible explanation for Cushing's syndrome associated with adrenal hyperplasia. J Clin Endocrinol Metab 20:1259–1268
O'Hare MJ, Hornsby PJ (1974) Absence of circadian rhythm of corticosterone secretion in monolayer cultures of adult rat adrenocortical cells. Experientia 31:378–380
Pearse AGE, Takor TT (1976) Neuroendocrine embryology and the APUD concept. Clin Endocrinol 5 (Suppl): 229s–244s
Pelletier G, Leclerc R, Labrie F, Cote J, Chretien M, Lis M (1977) Immunohistochemical localization of $\beta$-lipotropic hormone in the pituitary gland. Endocrinology 100:777–776
Pelletier G, Puviani R, Leclerc R (1979) Immunoelectron microscopic localization of ACTH, $\beta$-LPH and a fragment (16K) of their common precursor in rat brain. Prog. Endocrine Soc., 61st Meeting (Abstract)
Pelletier G, Robert F, Hardy J (1978) Identification of human anterior pituitary cells by immunoelectron microscopy. J Clin Endocrinol Metab 46:534–542

Phifer RF, Orth DN, Spicer SS (1974) Specific demonstration of the human hypophyseal adreno-cortico-melanotropic (ACTH/MSH) cell. J Clin Endocrinol Metab 39:684–692

Piezzi RS, Larin F, Wurtman RJ (1970) Serotonin, 5-hydroxyindoleacetic acid (5-HIAA) and monoamine oxidase in the bovine median eminence and pituitary gland. Endocrinology 86:1460–1462

Raisman G (1970) An evaluation of the basic pattern of connections between the limbic system and the hypothalamus. Am J Anat 129:197–202

Ratter SJ, Lowry PJ, Besser GM, Rees LH (1980) Chromatographic characterization of adreno-corticotrophin in human plasma. J Endocrinol 85:359–369

Roberts JL, Herbert E (1977) Characterization of a common precursor to corticotropin and $\beta$-lipotropin: Identification of $\beta$-lipotropin peptides and their arrangement relative to cortico-tropin in the precursor synthesized in a cell-free system. Proc Natl Acad Sci USA 74: 5300–5304

Roberts JL, Phillips M, Rosa PA, Herbert E (1978) Steps involved in the processing of common precursor forms of adrenocorticotropin and endorphin in cultures of mouse pituitary cells. Am Chem Soc 17:3609–3618

Rubinstein M, Stein S, Udenfriend S (1978) Characterization of pro-opiocortin, a precursor to opioid peptides and corticotropin. Proc Natl Acad Sci USA 75 (2):669–671

Saffran M, Schally AV, Benfey BG (1955) Stimulation of the release of corticotropin from the adenohypophysis by a neurohypophyseal factor. Endocrinology 57:439–444

Schally AV, Anderson RN, Lipscomb HS, Long JM, Guillemin R (1960) Evidence for the existence of two corticotrophin-releasing factors, $\alpha$ and $\beta$. Nature 188:1192–1193

Schwyzer R (1964) Chemistry and metabolic action of nonsteroid hormones. Ann Rev Biochem 33:259–286

Scott AP, Lowry PJ (1974) Adrenocorticotrophic and melanocyte-stimulating peptides in the human pituitary. Biochem J 139:593–602

Simon ML, George R (1975) Diurnal variations in plasma corticosterone and growth hormone as correlated with regional variations in norepinephrine, dopamine and serotonin content of rat brain. Neuroendocrinology 17:125–138

Siperstein ER, Miller KJ (1973) Hypertrophy of the ACTH-producing cell following adrenalec-tomy: A quantitative electron microscopic study. Endocrinology 93:1257–1268

Sirett NE, Gibbs FP (1969) Dexamethasone suppression of ACTH release: Effect of the interval between steroid administration and the application of stimuli known to release ACTH. Endo-crinology 85:355–359

Slusher MA (1964) Effects of chronic hypothalamic lesions on diurnal and stress corticosteroid levels. Am J Physiol 206: 1161–1164

Smelik PG (1963) Relation between blood level of corticoids and their inhibiting effect on the hypophyseal stress response. Proc Soc Exp Biol Med 113:616–619

Srivasian AK, Meier AH (1972) Daily variation in concentration of cortisol in plasma in intact and hypophysectomized Gulf killfish. Science 177:185–187

Suda T, Liotta AS, Krieger DT (1978) $\beta$-Endorphin is not detectable in plasma from normal human subjects. Science 202 (4364): 221–223

Takebe K, Kunita H, Sakukura M (1968) Effect of dexamethasone on ACTH release induced by lysine vasopressin in man: Time interval between dexamethasone and vasopressin injec-tion. J Clin Endocrinol 28:644–650

Takebe K, Kunita H, Sakukura M (1971) Suppressive effect of dexamethasone on the rise of CRF activity in the median eminence induced by stress. Endocrinology 89:1014–1019

Takebe K, Sakakura M, Mashimo K (1972) Continuance of diurnal rhythmicity of CRF activity in hypophysectomized rats. Endocrinology 90:1515–1520

Tanaka K, Nicholson WE, Orth DN (1978) The nature of the immunoreactive lipotropins in human plasma and tissue extract. J Clin Invest 62:94–104

Tyrrell JB, Lorenzi M, Forsham PH, Gerich JE (1975) The effect of somatostatin on secretion of adrenocorticotropin in normal subjects and in patients with Nelson's syndrome and Cushing's disease. Endocrine Soc, 57th Ann Meeting, vol 350, p 599 (Abstract)

Ungar F, Halberg F (1926) Circadian rhythm in the in vitro response of mouse adrenal to adreno-corticotrophic hormone. Science 137:1058–1059

Vale W, Rivier C (1977) Substances modulating the secretion of ACTH by cultured anterior pituitary cells. Fed Proc 36:2094–2099

Vale W, Spiess J, Rivier C, Rivier J (1981) Characterization of a 41-residue ovine hypothalamic peptide that stimulates secretion of corticotropin and β-endorphin. Science 213:1394–1397
Voigt KH, Fehm HL, Lang RE, Walter R (1976) The effect of somatostatin and of prolyl-leucyl-glycinamide (MIF) on ACTH release in dispersed pituitary cells. Life Sci 21:739–746
Yasuda N, Greer MA (1976) Distribution of corticotropin-releasing factor(s) activity in neural and extraneural tissues of the rat. Endocrinology 99:944–948
Yasuda N, Greer MA, Greer SE, Panton P (1977) Distribution of corticotropin releasing factor activity within the hypothalamic pituitary complex of rats and cattle. J Endocrinol 75:293–303
Yates FE, Maran JW (1974) Stimulation and inhibition of adrenocorticotropin release. In: Knobil E, Sawyer W (eds) Handbook of physiology. Am. Physiol Soc Washington, D.C., pp 367–404
Yasuda N, McClung M, Greer MA (1978) Demonstration of "big" CRF (corticotrophin-releasing factor) in bovine hypophyseal stalk. Biochem Biophys Res Commun 81:1187–1194
Zimmerman E, Critchlow V (1969a) Effects of intracerebral dexamethasone on pituitary-adrenal function in female rats. Am J Physiol 217:392–396
Zimmerman E, Critchlow V (1969b) Negative feedback and pituitary-adrenal function in female cats. Am J Physiol 216:148–155
Zimmerman EA, Stillman MA, Recht LD, Antunes JL, Carmel PW (1977) Vasopressin and corticotropin-releasing factor: An axonal pathway to portal capillaries in the zona externa of the median eminence containing vasopressin and its interaction with adrenal corticoids. In: Krieger DT, Ganong WF (eds) ACTH and related peptides: Structure, regulation and action. NY Acad Sci USA 207:405–419

*Chapter 3*

# ACTH Action

## A. Structure-Function Relationships

ACTH$^{1-39}$ has a multitude of actions, both on the adrenals and at extra-adrenal sites. Considerable effort has been expended in attempts to determine the structural sequences for these actions and the mechanisms by which they produce their effects. Most of the structure-function relationships have dealt with the steroidogenic activity of ACTH (Hofmann 1974; Schwyzer 1977). The concept has evolved that there are sequences which comprise the "active" or "message" site and the "attachment" or "address" site. The active site is contained within the 1–10 amino acid sequence, and the attachment site within the 9–18 amino acid sequence (Ontjes et al. 1977). ACTH$^{1-24}$ possesses biological activity equivalent to that of ACTH$^{1-39}$. The lesser activity of sequences comprising ACTH$^{1-19}$ through ACTH$^{1-23}$ is believed to be secondary, not to lessened receptor affinity but to an enhanced rate of degradation. Peptide sequences smaller than 1–18 exhibit markedly diminished activity. The C-terminal 25–39 appears to influence the degradation of the molecule, so that human 1–39 has a longer duration of action than 1–24 (Baumann and Felber, 1976).

It is also agreed that the earliest event in ACTH action is its interaction with a specific membrane receptor, leading to activation of membrane adenylcyclase and the formation within the cell of adenosine 3′:5′-cyclic phosphate (cAMP) which serves as the "second messenger" for ACTH action. There is some evidence that the potency of several ACTH analogs in stimulating cAMP production correlates with their steroidogenic potency. It also appears that the adrenal membrane possesses an excess of functional receptor-adenylcyclase complexes, over and above the number needed to induce maximum steroidogenesis. The reasons for this are unknown. Recent evidence suggests (Schulster and Breslow 1980) that there indeed may be two populations of ACTH receptors, occupancy of one being related to steroidogenesis and of the other to cAMP production. It is probable that ACTH also acts on the high-density lipoprotein (HDL) recognition site that governs substrate uptake. It has been shown that 80% or more of the cholesterol substrate for steroidogenesis comes from plasma. Uptake of lipoprotein-bound cholesterol is stimulated by ACTH, although there appears to be species variation as to whether HDL or LDL serves as the donor of extracellular cholesterol to the adrenal cell (Gwynn et al. 1978; Kovanen et al. 1979; Simpson and Carr 1979). Calcium may also act as a second messenger for ACTH. This appears to be required in the step between hormone-receptor binding and adenylate cyclase activation. It is believed to act by increasing the rate of activation by guanosine triphosphate (GTP) of an active conformation of the cyclase (Ontjes 1980).

## B. Effect on Adrenal Size, Morphology, and Growth

The increase in adrenal size produced by ACTH administration provided the basis for the first bioassay of this hormone. Such increase in size results from a combination of initial cell hypertrophy with a subsequent increase in cell number (Deane 1962). Morphologically, this is accompanied by enlargement of zona fasciculata cells, increased nuclear and nucleolar size, and increased numbers of mitochondria (Miller 1953; Miller 1954). The foregoing events have been observed after in vivo administration of natural ACTH and are accompanied by stimulation of DNA synthesis and activation of DNA polymerase (Saez et al. 1977). In vitro studies, however, have yielded opposite results. In experiments with cultured adrenocortical cells derived from either normal or tumorous adrenal tissue, it has been shown that ACTH inhibits cell replication (Masui and Garren 1971; Ramachandran and Suyama 1975), associated with inhibition of DNA synthesis (Ramachandran and Suyama 1975; Weidman and Gill 1977). It is believed that such inhibition is mediated by ACTH-induced generation of corticosteroids (Gospodarowicz and Gospodarowicz 1975) or of cAMP, the latter of which is also inhibitory to adrenal cell growth (Pastan et al. 1975).

At present, the reason for the discrepancy between in vivo and in vitro results is not clear. It may be that in vitro the increased intracellular accumulation of both cAMP and glucocorticoids following ACTH administration induces inhibition of DNA synthesis, while in the in vivo situation the release of both cAMP and glucocorticoids into the bloodstream prevents their accumulation and potential inhibition of cell growth. It should be noted that, even in vitro, after an initial period of inhibition of cell growth, "desensitization" to the effect of ACTH occurs and cells ultimately begin to grow despite the continued presence of ACTH (Hornsby and Gill 1977).

It has also been suggested that ACTH may induce the presence or delivery of growth factors to adrenal cortical cells, these factors being the actual stimuli of adrenal cell growth and proliferation. Candidates for such growth factors include angiotensin, insulin (Ramachandran and Suyama 1975), growth hormone (Cater and Stack-Dunne 1955), an uncharacterized adrenal weight-maintaining factor (Segal and Christy 1968), and fibroblast growth factor (Gospodarowicz et al. 1977). It should be noted that a fibroblast growth-factor-like molecule has been isolated from the pituitary (Jones and Gospodarowicz 1974), but no studies have been performed with regard to physiological regulation of such a factor. Additional support for the concept that non-ACTH factors are involved in adrenal growth is provided by reports that neural stimulation of the adrenal appears to result in growth by an ACTH-independent mechanism (Engeland and Dallman 1975) and that animals treated in vivo with ACTH antiserum show a significant decrease in serum corticosterone levels, which does not affect adrenal weight or the ability of such animals to increase adrenal weight, cell number, and DNA content of the remaining adrenal gland following unilateral adrenalectomy (Ramachandran and Suyama 1975).

## C. Mechanism of ACTH Action of Steroidogenesis

The first step in ACTH action consists of binding to specific receptors in adrenal cell membranes (Hofmann et al. 1970; Lefkowitz et al. 1971; Saez et al. 1974; Ways et al. 1976). This results in activation of plasma-membrane-bound adenylate cyclase, with a resultant increase in intracellular cAMP concentrations (Grahame-Smith et al. 1967; Taunton et al. 1969). cAMP next binds to a regulatory subunit of cyclic AMP protein kinase and liberates the fully activated catalytic subunit, which then phosphorylates several intracellular protein substrates that may represent rate-limiting steps in steroidogenesis (Garren et al. 1971; Walton and Gill 1977).

The nature of this (these) postulated protein(s) is not known. It is believed that such proteins act at the site whereby ACTH stimulates steroidogenesis, namely, the conversion of cholesterol to pregnenolone via side-chain cleavage of cholesterol. Such a protein would have a rapid turnover time, in view of the speedy decline in cortisol secretion following removal of ACTH. Additional support for the concept that ACTH action is mediated by a protein is provided by reports that cyclohexamide (Davis and Garren 1968) and puromycin (Ferguson 1963) block the steroidogenic action of ACTH and cAMP. Actinomycin-D, which blocks RNA synthesis, has no effect on the steroidogenic action of ACTH (Ferguson and Morita 1965). Since the effect of ACTH is seen so quickly (i.e., 3 min after administration), Koritz et al. (1977) have suggested that, rather than synthesis of a protein being involved in ACTH action, the effect of ACTH in increasing the concentration of cAMP regulates the extent to which such a rapidly turning-over protein is converted (via phosphorylation) to an active form, which can then stimulate conversion of cholesterol to pregnenolone, perhaps by inducing increasing binding of cholesterol to side-chain cleavage P450 (Alfano et al. 1973; Brownie and Alfano 1973). It is postulated that this rapidly turning-over protein may be present in excess and that the concentration of the active form will depend only on the extent of activation of the appropriate protein kinase by ACTH. In the presence of protein synthesis inhibitors, however, the level of this protein can drop to a point where it becomes rate-limiting. Another report characterizes a protein whose concentration is significantly increased 2 h following ACTH administration, this peptide representing approximately 10% of the total protein synthesis induced by ACTH via cAMP (Dazord et al. 1977).

Other studies, however, indicate that under proper conditions, inhibition of protein synthesis does not affect stimulation of steroidogenesis by ACTH and cAMP, i.e., that at low concentration of protein synthesis inhibitors the inhibition of protein synthesis is considerably greater than that of steroidogenesis (Koritz et al. 1957; Kowal 1970). There is, therefore, controversy as to whether ACTH acts by increasing a specific protein (Dazord et al. 1977) or, as Koritz suggests, by increasing the activation of a previously present protein.

Another role that has been suggested for ACTH (Haynes and Berthet 1957) is that of activation of adrenal phosphorylase via cAMP, leading to an increase in glycogenolysis and glucose metabolism via the hexose monophosphate shunt, with resultant increases in nicotanamide adenine dinucleotide phosphate, reduced form (NADPH). This could then act as a source of reducing equivalents in the cytochrome P450 system of steroid hydroxylation (see Chap. 4). Still another effect of ACTH is inhibition of 5$\alpha$-reductase activity (Kitay et al. 1971). This results in greater adrenal corticosteroid output by diminishing the formation of reduced metabolites. Growth hormone and prolactin have been reported to lower the elevated 5$\alpha$-reductase activities seen in hypophysectomized rats (Colby et al. 1973; Witorsch and Kitay 1972). This may be physiologically significant, since adrenal prolactin binding sites and growth hormone binding sites have been demonstrated (Posner et al. 1974). Androgens have also been reported to have a direct effect in decreasing 5$\alpha$-reductase activity (Colby and Kitay 1972), whereas a similar effect of estrogen may be mediated via enhanced ACTH or prolactin secretion.

The prostaglandins $PGE_1$ and $PGE_2$ have also been reported to increase adrenal steroidogenesis. The significance of the specific receptors for these prostaglandins that have been demonstrated in human adrenal glands (Dazord and Saez 1978) remains to be explored. These are presumably different from the receptors that bind ACTH, although both sets of receptors effect activation of adenylate cyclase.

## D. Effect of ACTH on Aldosterone Secretion

Although the basic mechanisms of ACTH elevation of corticosteroidogenesis apply to aldosterone, it appears that there are factors other than ACTH that regulate such secretion. It is agreed that ACTH causes prompt short-term increases in aldosterone secretion (Biglieri et al. 1969; Ganong et al. 1966). Such secretion, however, is stimulated only by doses of ACTH exceeding those required to achieve maximal corticosteroidogenesis. After several days of treatment with large doses of ACTH, aldosterone levels fall to normal or low values. This is believed to be secondary to a compensatory reduction in renin release as a result of aldosterone-induced expansion of extracellular fluid volume. This is compatible with other findings which indicate that the renin-angiotensin system is a major regulator of aldosterone production (Kaplan and Bartter 1962), angiotensin also stimulating conversion of cholesterol to pregnenolone.

## E. Dynamics of ACTH Secretion

Consideration of ACTH action should involve cognizance of its distribution within the body fluids and its disappearance, as well as the dose-response characteristics of its effect on the adrenal. It is controversial as to whether circulating ACTH is bound to plasma proteins(s) (Upton et al. 1970). Estimates of the half-life of immunoreactive ACTH in the human vary from 17 to 30 min (Berson and Yalow 1968; Liotta et al. 1978). Such disappearance appears to be biphasic. The half-life of bioactive ACTH is much shorter, approximately 2–3 min (Nicholson et al. 1978), and appears to follow a single exponential function. The volume of ACTH distribution appears to be 10–20%

of body weight (Liotta et al. 1978). Its metabolic clearance rate varies between 0.2–0.3 liter/min at physiological concentrations; rates of 1.3 liter/min have been reported at high rates of ACTH infusion (Liddle et al. 1962). The greatest amounts of tissue uptake occur in kidney, liver, muscle, skin, gastrointestinal tract, and adipose tissue. Degradation occurs within these tissues; in addition, the kidney irreversibly clears the parent peptide and its peptide fragments (Bennet and McMartin 1979). However, the only organ to demonstrate a specific uptake mechanism is the adrenal (Nicholson et al. 1978). It is believed that ACTH may be catabolized within lysosomes following tissue uptake. The nature of the fragments produced, whether they circulate, and whether they might act competitively at the ACTH receptor, preventing further ACTH action, remain to be determined.

There is virtually no delay in the adrenal corticosteroid response to ACTH. Several generalizations can be made about this reponse. The total magnitude and duration of the response are directly proportional to the dose of ACTH. The greater the dose administered over a given time period, the greater the height and duration of the adrenal corticosteroidogenic response. The initial rate of rise in plasma cortisol concentrations in response to varying doses of ACTH is the same (McDonald et al. 1969). There is an approximately linear relationship between plasma corticosteroid concentration and that of the logarithm of plasma ACTH concentration from approximately 5–300 pg/ml (Ney et al. 1963). Beyond this concentration, further increments in ACTH dosage do not induce further increments in cortisol secretion (Fig. 3.1). Tachyphylaxis has also been observed; repeated treatment with ACTH (i.e., within a 1–2-day period) results in a greater response to a given dose on the second

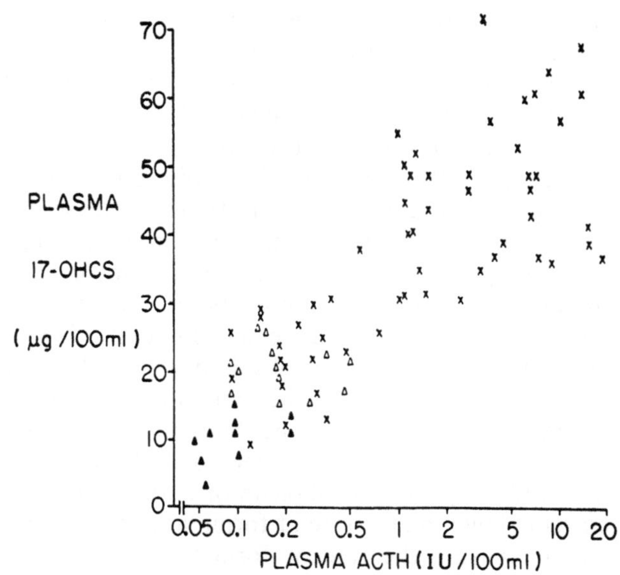


**Fig. 3.1.** Each point represents a coordinate value for simultaneous plasma ACTH and 17-OHCS concentrations in normal subjects: 6 PM (▲); 6 AM (△); subjects receiving ACTH infusions (×). From Ney et al. (1963) with permission

occasion of presentation. A given dose of ACTH stimulates greater amounts of corticosteroid secretion when it is given over a longer period of time (Eik-Nes et al. 1954). This may in part reflect the contribution of previously secreted cortisol (with its approximately 70-min half-life) to the final corticosteroid concentration observed at the end of the time span studied. When ACTH concentration is kept constant, but the duration of administration varies, the total amount of corticosteroid secreted in the different time spans is the same. As an example of the effects of dose versus concentration, $\chi$ units of ACTH infused i.v. over a 5-h period stimulates a smaller increase in corticosteroids than the same dose infused over a 10- or 20-h period. However, if the adrenals are exposed to $2\chi$ units/ml for 60 min, or $60\chi$ units/ml for 2 min, an equal amount of cortisol is secreted over a 90-min period (Urquhart 1974). Finally, the temporal pattern of ACTH presentation also governs adrenal response. Such considerations are important in view of the demonstrated episodic nature of ACTH release (Krieger and Allen 1975). If the frequency of ACTH presentation is increased beyond one cycle per 10 min, the glands' sinusoidal secretory response does not follow. Therefore, if the mean ACTH concentration is kept constant within a relatively small range, but the frequency of presentation to the adrenal over a finite time span varies, greater corticosteroid secretion will occur at the lower frequency, i.e., there is less secretion with one cycle for 5 min than with one cycle for 20 min (Fig. 3.2).

## F. Extra-adrenal Metabolic Actions of ACTH

One of the most prominent extra-adrenal actions of ACTH is its rapidly occurring lipolytic effect. There is, however, no extensive study to determine whether such an effect occurs in vivo within the physiological range of ACTH concentrations. Infusion of ACTH at 10 units/h, which is the maximal rate of endogenous ACTH release as seen in patients with secondary adrenal insufficiency (Stamp et al. 1965), did not result in any lipolytic effect. In in vitro perfusion experiments, fatty acid release can be stimulated by ACTH, but again with concentrations well beyond the upper limit of the physiological range in plasma (Scow et al. 1965). Similar reservations pertain regarding the nonphysiological nature of the dose of ACTH reported to produce hypoglycemia and hyperinsulinemia (Lebovitz 1965). The single extra-adrenal effect that appears to be physiological is the effect of ACTH in increasing melanin pigmentation of the skin (Lerner and McGuire 1964). This activity is probably secondary to the 7-amino acid sequence ($ACTH^{4-10}$) common to the intact ACTH molecule and to $\alpha$-MSH. ACTH has also been shown to alter the peripheral metabolism of cortisol, increasing the half-life of injected cortisol, lowering the rate of formation of glucuronide conjugated metabolites, and increasing the rate of formation of $6\beta$-hydroxycortisol and of sulfate conjugated metabolites. This has been interpreted as secondary to an effect of ACTH in inhibiting enzyme response for ring A reduction and perhaps for $11\beta$-OH dehydrogenation (Kornel 1970).

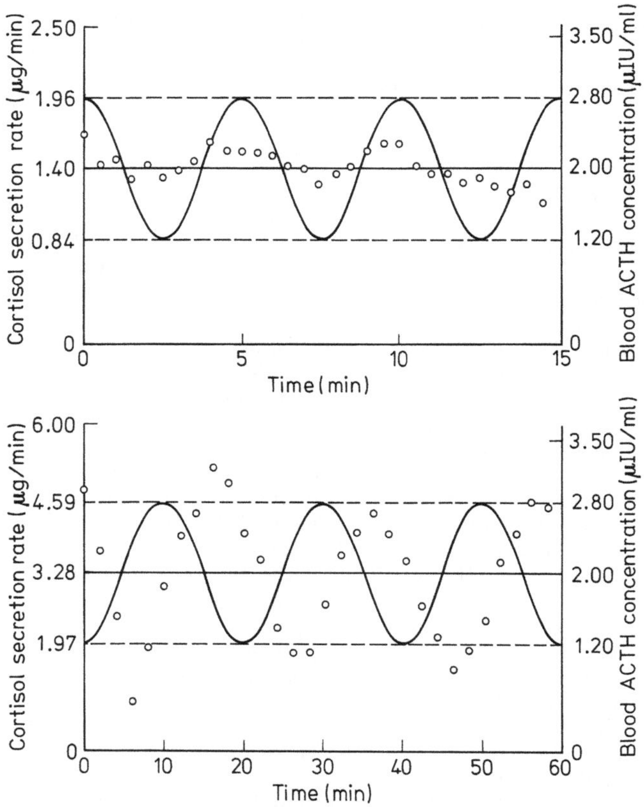


**Fig. 3.2.** Time course of cortisol secretion rate *(points)* during sinusoidal variations in ACTH concentration *(line)* at 0.2 cycles per minute *(upper figure)* or 0.05 cycles per minute *(lower figure).* Zero time corresponds to minute 60 of sinusoidal stimulation. The two *ordinate scales* in each figure are related, assuming that the increment in cortisol secretion rate above the residual value (ACTH = 0) is linearly related to ACTH concentration of 0 to at least 3 μIU ACTH/ml. With 0.2 cycles per minute, the residual secretion rate (ACTH = 0) was 0.29 μg/min, the secretory maximum of this gland was 11.8 μg/min, whereas with 0.05 cycles per minute the residual secretion rate was 0.06 μg/min and the maximum secretion rate was 10.9 μg/min. It can be seen that the glands' sinusoidal response dissipates as frequency of stimulation increases. From Urquhart (1974) with permission

## G. Behavioral Effects of ACTH

There are numerous reports that, in the rat, ACTH and ACTH fragments have marked effects on learning and behavior in the absence of the pituitary or the adrenals (de Wied 1974). The smallest effective fragment with regard to learning is the 4–7 sequence of the ACTH molecule; effects on memory can also be elicited with the 4–10 fragment. Inconsistent results have been reported in human studies. There is also a report that ACTH and ACTH fragments enhance (within a critical period) CNS maturation (van der Helm-Hylkema and de Wied 1976). The molecular basis of these neural and behavioral effects is unknown. $ACTH^{4-10}$ does increase catecholamine turnover and synthesis in brains of intact rats, but does not do so in hypophysectomized or adrenalectomized animals, where it is also behaviorally effective (Versteeg and Wurtman 1975).

## References


Alfano JA, Brownie AC, Orme-Johnson WH, Beinert H (1973) Adrenal mitochondrial cytochrome P-450 and cholesterol side chain cleavage activity. J Biol Chem 248:7860–7864

Baumann G, Felber J-P (1976) Prolonged corticotropin action of synthetic human ACTH in man. J Clin Endocrinol Metab 42:160–163

Bennett HPJ, McMartin C (1979) Distribution and degradation of two tritium-labelled corticotropin analogues in the rat. J Endocrinol 82:33–42

Berson SA, Yalow RS (1968) Radioimmunoassay of ACTH in plasma. J Clin Invest 47:2725–2751

Besser G, Orth DN, Nicholson WE (1971) Dissociation of the disappearance of bioactive and radioimmunoreactive ACTH from plasma in man. J Clin Endocrinol 32:595–603

Biglieri EG, Schambelan M, Slaton PE Jr (1969) Effect of adrenocorticotropin on deoxycorticosterone, corticosterone and aldosterone excretion. J Clin Endocrinol Metab 29:1090–1101

Brownie AC, Alfano J (1973) Effect of ACTH on adrenal mitochondrial cytochrome P-450 in the rat. Ann NY Acad Sci 212:344–360

Cater DB, Stack-Dunne MP (1955) The effects of growth hormone and corticotrophin upon the adrenal, weight and adrenocortical mitotic activity in the hypophysectomized rat. J Endocrinol 12:174–184

Colby HD, Caffrey JL, Kitay JI (1973) Interaction of growth hormone and ACTH in the regulation of adrenocortical secretion in rats. Endocrinology 93:188–192

Colby HD, Kitay JI (1972) Effects of gonadal hormones on adrenal cortical secretion of 5$\alpha$-reduced metabolites of corticosterone in the rat. Endocrinology 91:1523–1527

Davis WW, Garren LD (1968) On the mechanism of action of adrenocorticotropic hormone. J Biol Chem 243: 5153–5157

Dazord A, Gallet D, Saez JM (1977) ACTH-dependent stimulation of a specific peptide in adrenocortical cells in culture. Biochem Biophys Res Commun 76:1238–1246

Dazord A, Saez JM (1978) ACTH and prostaglandin receptors in human adrenocortical tumors. In: James VHT, Serio M, Giusti G, Martini L (eds) The endocrine function of the human adrenal cortex. Academic Press, New York, pp 123–136

Deane HW (1962) The anatomy, chemistry, and physiology of adrenocortical tissue. In: Deane HW (ed) Handbuch der Experimentellen Pharmakologie. The adrenal hormones, their origin, chemistry, physiology and pharmacology. Springer, Berlin Göttingen Heidelberg, pp 1–185

DeWied D (1974) Pituitary-adrenal system: Hormones and behavior. In: Schmitt FO, Worden FG (eds) The neurosciences third study program. MIT Press, Cambridge, Mass., pp 653–666

Eik-Nes K, Sandberg AA, Nelson DH (1954) Changes in plasma levels of 17-hydroxycorticosteroids during the intravenous administration of ACTH. I. A test of adrenocortical capacity in the human. J Clin Invest 33:1502–1508

Engeland WC, Dallman MF (1975) Compensatory adrenal growth is neurally mediated. Neuroendocrinology 19:352–362

Ferguson JJ Jr (1963) Protein synthesis and adrenocorticotropin responsiveness. J Biol Chem 238:2754–2759

Ferguson JJ Jr, Morita Y (1965) RNA synthesis and adrenocorticotropin responsiveness. Biochem Biophys Acta 87:348–350

Ganong WF, Biglieri EG, Mulrow PJ (1966) Mechanisms regulating adrenocortical secretion of aldosterone and glucocorticoids. Recent Prog Horm Res 22:381–414

Garren LD, Gill GN, Masui H, Walton GM (1971) On the mechanism of action of ACTH. Recent Prog Horm Res 27:433–478

Gospodarowicz D, Gospodarowicz F (1975) The morphological transformation and inhibition of growth of bovine luteal cells in tissue culture induced by luteinizing hormone and dibutyryl cyclic AMP. Endocrinology 96:458–467

Gospodarowicz D, Ill CR, Hornsby PJ, Gill GN (1977) Control of bovine adrenal cortical cell proliferation by fibroblast growth factor. Lack of effect of epidermal growth factor. Endocrinology 100:1080–1089

Grahame-Smith G, Butcher RW, Ney RL, Sutherland EW (1967) Adenosine 3′,5′-monophosphate as the intracellular mediator of the action of adrenocorticotropic hormone on the adrenal cortex. J Biol Chem 242:5535–5541

Gwynne J, Hess B, Rountree R, Wolf W (1978) Enhancement of steroidogenesis by serum lipoproteins in human, rat and mouse adrenal cells. Endocrine Soc, 60th Ann Meeting, p 221 (Abstract)

Haynes RC Jr, Berthet L (1957) Studies on the mechanism of action of the adrenocorticotropic hormone. J Biol Chem 225:115–124

Helm-Hylkema van der H, de Wied D (1976) Effect of neonatally injected ACTH and ACTH analogues on eye-opening of the rat. Life Sci 18:1099–1104

Hofmann K (1974) Relations between chemical structure and function of adrenocorticotropin and melanocyte-stimulating hormones. In: Knobil E, Sawyer W (eds) Handbook of physiology, vol IV. American Physiological Society, Washington, D.C., p 29–58

Hofman K, Wingender W, Finn FM (1970) Correlation of adrenocorticotropic activity of ACTH analogs with degree of binding to an adrenal cortical particulate preparation. Proc Natl Acad Sci USA 67:829–836

Hornsby PJ, Gill GN (1977) Hormonal control of adrenocortical cell proliferation. J Clin Invest 60:342–352

Jones KL, Gospodarowicz D (1974) Biological activity of a growth factor for ovarian cells. Proc Natl Acad Sci USA 71:3372–3376

Kaplan NM, Bartter FC (1962) The effect of ACTH, renin, angiotensin II, and various precursors on biosynthesis of aldosterone by adrenal slices. J Clin Invest 41:715–724

Kitay JI, Coyne MD, Swygert NH, Gaines KE (1971) Effects of gonadal hormones and ACTH on the nature and rates of secretion of adrenocortical steroids by the rat. Endocrinology 89:565–570

Koritz SB, Bhargana, G, Schwartz E (1977) ACTH action on adrenal steroidogenesis. In: Krieger DT, Ganong WF (eds) ACTH and related peptides: Structure regulation, and action. NY Acad Sci 297:329–335

Koritz SM, Peron FG, Dorfman RI (1957) Influence of adrenocorticotropic hormone on corticoid production and glycine-1-$C^{14}$ incorporation into protein by rat adrenals. J Biol Chem 226:643–650

Kornel L: Corticosteroids in human blood. V. Extra-adrenal effect of ACTH upon metabolism of cortisol. In: Steroidologia No. 4, vol I. Karger, Basel, p 225–245

Kovanen PT, Faust JR, Brown MS, Goldstein JL (1979) Low density lipoprotein receptors in bovine adrenal cortex. I. Receptor-mediated uptake of low density lipoprotein and utilization of its cholesterol for steroid synthesis in cultured adrenocortical cells. Endocrinology 104: 599–609

Kowal J (1970) Adrenal cells in tissue culture. VII. Effect of inhibitors of protein synthesis on steroidogenesis and glycolysis. Endocrinology 87: 951–965

Krieger DT, Allen W (1975) Relationship of bioassayable and immunoassayable ACTH and cortisol concentrations in normal subjects and in patients with Cushing's disease. J Clin Endocrinol Metab 40:675–687

Lebovitz E, Bryant K, Frohman LA (1965) Acute effects of corticotropin and related peptides on carbohydrate and lipid metabolism. Ann NY Acad Sci 131:274–287

Lefkowitz RJ, Roth J, Pastan I (1971) ACTH-receptor interaction in the adrenal: A model for the initial step in the action of hormones that stimulate adenyl cyclase. Ann NY Acad Sci 185:195–209

Lerner AB, McGuire JS (1964) Melanocyte-stimulating hormone and adrenocorticotrophic hormone. N Engl J Med 270:539–546

Liddle GW, Island D, Meador CK (1962) Normal and abnormal regulation of corticotropin secretion in man. Recent Prog Horm Res 18:125–153

Liotta AS, Li CH, Schussler GC, Krieger DT (1978) Comparative metabolic clearance rate, volume of distribution and plasma half-life of human $\beta_h$-lipotropin and ACTH. Life Sci 23:2323–2330

Masui H, Garren LD (1971) Inhibition of replication in functional mouse adrenal tumor cells by adrenocorticotropic hormone mediated by adenosine 3′,5′-cyclic monophosphate. Proc Natl Acad Sci USA 68:3206–3210

McDonald RK, Sollberger AR, Mueller PS, Sheard MH (1969) The effect of small doses of human ACTH on serum corticosteroid levels in man. Proc Soc Exp Biol Med 131:1091–1094
Miller RA (1953) The relation of mitochondria to secretory activity in the fascicular zone of the rat's adrenal. Am J Anat 92:329–360
Ney RL, Shimizu N, Nicholson WE, Island DP, Liddle GW (1963) Correlation of plasma ACTH concentration with adrenocortical response in normal human subjects, surgical patients, and patients with Cushing's disease. J Clin Invest 42:1169–1167
Nicholson WE, Liddle RA, Puett D, Liddle GW (1978) Adrenocorticotropic hormone biotransformation, clearance, and catabolism. Endocrinology 103:1344–1351
Ontjes DA (1980) The pharmacologic control of adrenal steroidogenesis. Life Sci 26:2023–2035
Ontjes DA, Ways DK, Mahafee DD, Zimmerman CF, Gwynne JT (1977) ACTH receptors and the effect of ACTH on adrenal organelles. In: Krieger DT, Ganong WF (eds) ACTH and related peptides: Structure, regulation and action. NY Acad Sci 297:295–313
Pastan IH, Johnson GC, Anderson WB (1975) Role of cyclic nucleotide in growth control. Ann Rev Biochem 44:491–522
Posner BI, Kelly PA, Shiu RPC, Friesen HG (1974) Studies of insulin, growth hormone and prolactin binding: tissue distribution, species variation and characterization. Endocrinology 95:521–531
Ramachandran J, Suyama AT (1975) Inhibition of replication of normal adrenocortical cells in culture by adrenocorticotropin. Proc Natl Acad Sci USA 72:113–117
Saez JM, Morera AM, Dazord AM, Bataille P (1974) Interactions of ACTH with its adrenal receptors: Specific binding of $ACTH_{1-24}$, its 0-nitrophenyl sulfanyl derivative and $ACTH_{11-24}$. J Steroid Biochem 5:925–933
Saez JM, Morera AM, Gallet D (1977) Opposite effects of ACTH and glucocorticoids on adrenal DNA synthesis in vivo. Endocrinology 100:1268–1275
Schulster D, Breslow AF (1980) Biochemical and genetic analyses of ACTH mechanism of action. Proc. VI. Intl. Congr. Endocrinol, Melbourne, p 157 (Abstract)
Schwyzer R (1977) ACTH: A short introductory review. In: Krieger DT, Ganong WF (eds) ACTH and related peptides, Structure, regulation and action. NY Acad Sci 297:3–26
Scow RO, Sticker FA, Pick TY, Clary TR (1965) Effect of ACTH on FFA release and diglyceride content in rat adipose tissue. Ann NY Acad Sci 131:288–301
Segal BM, Christy NP (1968) Potentiation of the biologic activity of ACTH by human plasma. A preliminary study. J Clin Endocrinol 28:1456–1472
Simpson ER, Carr BR (1979) Metabolism of serum lipoproteins by the human fetal adrenal. Endocrine Soc, 61st Meeting, p 218 (Abstract)
Stamp TCB, Landon J, Wynn V (1965) Observations on some extra-adrenal effects of corticotropin on carbohydrate and lipid metabolism in man. Metabolism 14:1041–1050
Taunton OD, Roth J, Pastan I (1969) Studies on the adrenocorticotropic hormone-activated adenyl cyclase of a functional adrenal tumor. J Biol Chem 244:247–253
Upton GV, Hollingsworth DR, Lande S, Lerner AB, Amatruda TT Jr (1970) Comparison of purified human and porcine ACTH in man. J Clin Endocrinol Metab 30:190–195
Urquhart J (1974) Physiological actions of adrenocorticotrophic hormone. In: Knobil E, Sawyer W (eds) Handbook of physiology, vol IV. American Physiological Society, Washington, D.C, p 133–157
Versteeg DHG, Wurtman RJ (1975) Effect of $ACTH^{4-10}$ on the rate of synthesis of $[^3H]$ catecholamines in the brains of intact, hypophysectomized and adrenalectomized rats. Brain Res 93:552–557
Walton GM, Gill GN (1973) Adenosine 3′,5′-monophosphate and protein kinase dependent phosphorylation of ribosomal protein. Biochemistry 12:2604–2611
Ways DK, Zimmerman CF, Ontjes DA (1976) Inhibition of adrenocorticotropin effects on adrenal cell membranes by synthetic adrenocorticotropin analogues: Correlation of binding and adenylate cyclase activation. Molec Pharmacol 12:789–799
Weidman EF, Gill GN (1977) Differential effects of ACTH or 8-Br-cAMP on growth and replication in a functional adrenal tumor cell line. J Cell Physiol 90:91–103
Witorsch RJ, Kitay JI (1972) Pituitary hormones affecting adrenal $5\alpha$-reductase activity: ACTH, growth hormone, and prolactin. Endocrinology 91:764–769

*Chapter 4*

# Actions of Adrenocortical Hormones

The clinical and laboratory abnormalities seen in Cushing's disease can all be related to known physiological and pharmacological effects of glucocorticoid hormones[1], since, in cases of Cushing's disease and syndrome, glucocorticoid concentrations may rise well into the pharmacological range (Table 4.1). These hormones affect virtually all body tissues. In recent years, investigators have sought to establish a common basic mechanism for all glucocorticoid actions (Baxter and Forsham 1972). It is believed that both the catabolic and anabolic responses seen with corticosteroid administration reflect the expression of similar mechanisms in different tissues (Leung and Munck 1975). In tissues possessing glucocorticoid receptors, glucocorticoid

**Table 4.1.** Effects of glucocorticoids

| | | Side effects |
|---|---|---|
| *Actions on metabolism* | | |
| 1. Carbohydrate metabolism | | Hyperglycemia, glycosuria, secondary hyperinsulinism |
| Increased gluconeogenesis | Liver<br>Kidney | |
| Decreased cellular glucose uptake | | |
| Increased glycogen deposition | | |
| 2. Fat metabolism (on white fat only) | | Characteristic fat distribution |
| Decreased lipogenesis | | |
| Increased lypolysis | | |
| Increased glycerol, fatty acids | | |
| 3. Protein metabolism | | Muscle weakness and wasting, striae, osteoporosis, decreased wound healing |
| Increased catabolism<br>↑ Gluconeogenesis<br>Negative nitrogen balance | Skeletal<br>Muscle<br>Skin<br>Lymphoid tissue<br>Connective tissue, bone<br>Adipose tissue<br>(Note opposite effects in liver) | |
| Inhibition of amino acid transport | | |
| Decreased synthesis (i.e., collagen) | | |
| Decreased RNA polymerase | | |

Continued next page

1 Some degree of virilization is also frequently seen in cases of Cushing's disease, since adrenal androgen production is ACTH-dependent and may therefore be stimulated in the pituitary-dependent variety of Cushing's disease. Androgens may also be elevated in cases of adrenal adenoma and carcinoma. In these instances, acquired enzymatic blocks can result in accumulation and secretion of adrenal androgens, chiefly dehydroepiandrosterone, $\Delta^4$ androstenedione, and testosterone, the two former being only weakly androgenic

**Table 4.1** (continued)

| | Side effects |
|---|---|
| 4. Electrolyte and water flux | Edema, sodium retention |
| Increased free $H_2O$ clearance | |
| $Na^+$ rentention, $K^+$ loss (large doses) | |
| Depressed ADH release | |
| Decreased gastrointestinal $Ca^{++}$ absorption (via inhibition of 25 hydroxylation of calciferol) | |
| Increased urinary calcium excretion | |
| *Actions on specific tissues* | |
| 1. Blood cells | Thrombophlebitis |
| ↑ Neutrophils | |
| ↑ Platelets | |
| ↑ Erythrocytes | |
| ↓ Lymphocytes | |
| ↓ Eosinophils | |
| ↓ Basophils | |
| 2. Peripheral vascular | Hypertension |
| Potentiate pressor effects of catecholamines | |
| Increased hepatic production of angiotensinogen | |
| 3. Central nervous system | Sleeplessness, mood changes, psychosis |
| Possible effects on enzymes involved in neurotransmitter synthesis (i.e., serotonin) | |
| Alteration in thresholds of electrical excitability and of sensory perception | |
| 4. Stomach | Peptic ulcer |
| Increase in stimulated gastric secretion | |
| High doses inhibit cell growth | |
| 5. Lung | |
| Induction of surfactant production in fetal lung | |
| *Actions on body processes* | |
| 1. Immune system | |
| High doses suppress certain antibody responses | Increase susceptibility to infection |
| Lymphocyte cytolysis or growth inhibition | |
| Suppresses cell-mediated immune response | |
| Thymus regression | |
| 2. Inflammatory response | |
| Inhibit phagocytic mechanisms | |
| Inhibit kinin release | |
| *Actions on other hormones* | |
| ↑ Prolactin | Galactorrhea |
| ↓ Growth hormone release | Growth retardation |
| ↓ TSH release | |
| ↓ Gonadotropin release | |
| ↓ ACTH release | |

action is mediated via steroid receptor interaction (see below) (Rousseau 1978). In other tissues lacking these receptors, such action may be mediated by mechanisms that involve membrane interactions. In certain instances, steroids have a direct effect on the processes that they affect. In others, their role has been described as "permissive," i.e., being necessary to effect the expression of other substances (see below).

## A. Pathways of Corticosteroid Biosynthesis

Figure 4.1 indicates the generally accepted pathway of corticosteroid biosynthesis. The hydroxylations depicted as occurring in steps *3, 7,* and *8* take place in mitochondria and involve oxidation of NADPH and steroids. The enzymes involved are called mixed-function oxidases. As shown in Fig. 4.2, cholesterol, indicated as steroid (S), is bound to cytochrome P450, enabling it to accept two electrons donated by reduced adrenodoxin, an iron-sulfur protein. Cholesterol is thus hydroxylated and pregnenolone released. Oxygen for the reaction is derived from molecular oxygen, which is activated by cytochrome P450 to form the superoxide ion $.O_2^-$ and peroxy ion $.O_2^{2-}$ (Fig. 4.2). This system, therefore, provides the terminal oxidase, which is in some way related to the desmolase that catalyzes the final carbon–carbon bond cleavage. Although the scheme for mitochondrial hydroxylation at the 11-$\beta$ and -18 position involves the same type of terminal oxidase, there is good evidence for the existence of different species of cytochrome P450 for these reactions. It is uncertain how cholesterol gets into mitochondria, and the indicated sequences of hydroxylation, oxidation, and C–C bond fission have not been completely confirmed. The steroid hydroxylations depicted in Fig. 4.1, steps *6* and *5a*, take place in smooth endoplasmic reticulum (SER) and differ from those occurring in mitochondria, in that these membranes do not contain the iron-sulfur protein (adrenodoxin) as seen in mitochondria.

## B. Mechanism of Glucocorticoid Action

It is believed that the molecular basis of glucocorticoid action is similar in virtually all glucocorticoid-sensitive tissues. This consists of entry of the steroid into the cell and its binding to a specific intracellular receptor protein. It is thought that such a receptor protein can exist in two conformations; active and inactive. Those steroids that act as agonists would bind to and stabilize the active conformation, while those that act as antagonists would bind and stabilize the inactive conformation. Such an inactive conformation cannot elicit a steroidogenic response. The affinity constants of different steroid analogs are in keeping with their known glucocorticoid activity. Although it is believed that the physicochemical properties of the glucocorticoid receptors are similar, if not identical in different tissues and in different species, some questions are raised by the observation that the relative potency of glucocorticoids varies in different target tissues, and that in some instances a steroid may act as an antagonist and in others as agonist (Rousseau et al. 1972).

Once the steroid has bound to the receptor protein, this complex undergoes a form of "activation," in part dependent on temperature and ionic strength. In some way, this enables the protein steroid complex to enter the nucleus and bind to nuclear chromatin. The steroid specificity for nuclear binding is the same as that for the cytosol receptor. Such nuclear binding is in some manner able to effect the appearance of increased mRNA for the specific

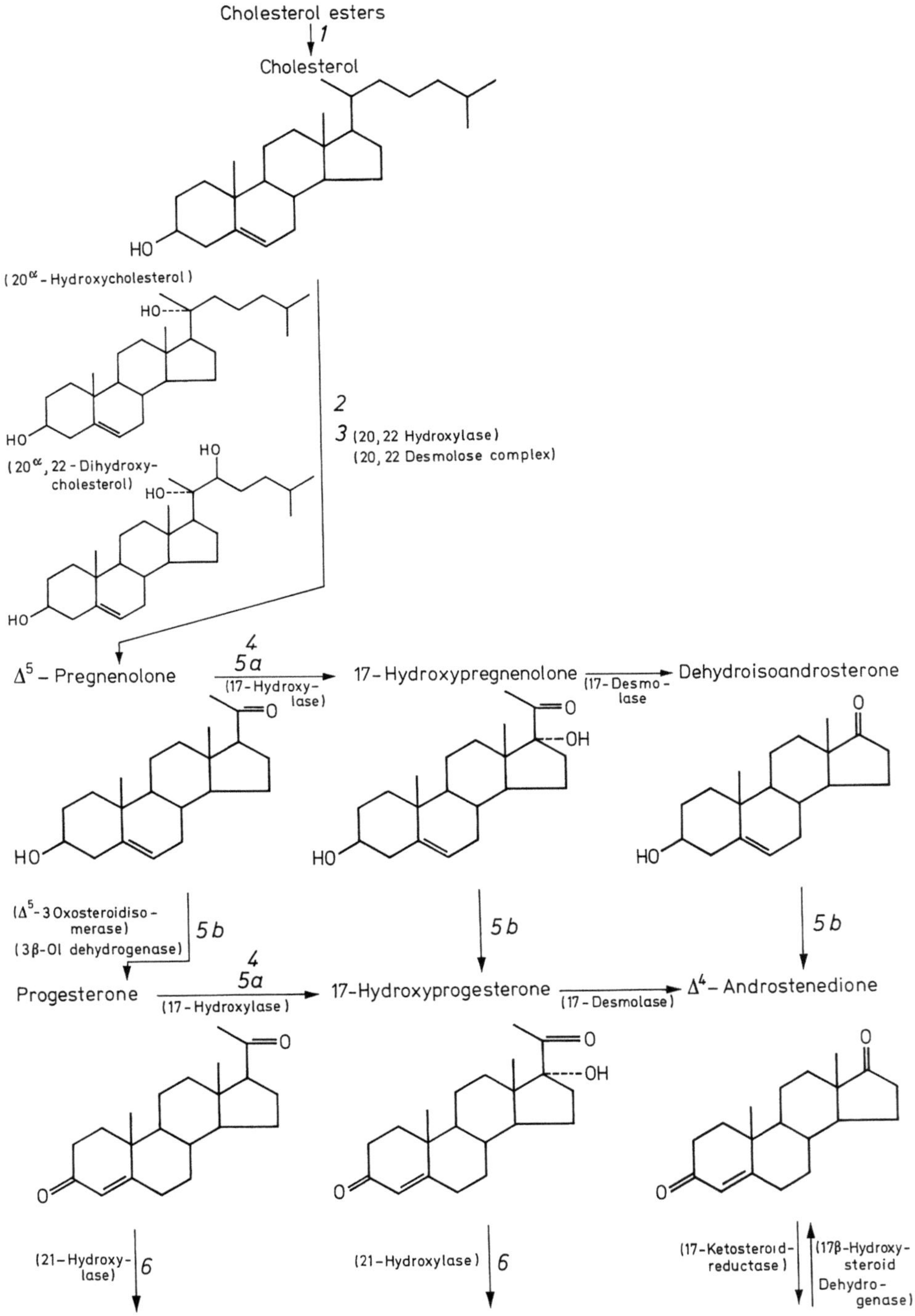
Cholesterol esters
1
Cholesterol
HO
(20α - Hydroxycholesterol)
HO
HO
2
3 (20, 22 Hydroxylase)
(20, 22 Desmolose complex)
(20α, 22 - Dihydroxy-cholesterol)
HO
HO
HO
Δ5 - Pregnenolone
4
5a
(17-Hydroxy-lase)
17-Hydroxypregnenolone
(17-Desmo-lase
Dehydroisoandrosterone
O
O
OH
O
HO
HO
HO
(Δ5-3 Oxosteroidiso-merase)
(3β-Ol dehydrogenase)
5b
5b
5b
Progesterone
4
5a
(17-Hydroxylase)
17-Hydroxyprogesterone
(17-Desmolase)
Δ4- Androstenedione
O
O
OH
O
O
O
O
(21-Hydroxy-lase)
6
(21-Hydroxylase)
6
(17-Ketosteroid-reductase)
(17β-Hydroxy-steroid Dehydro-genase)

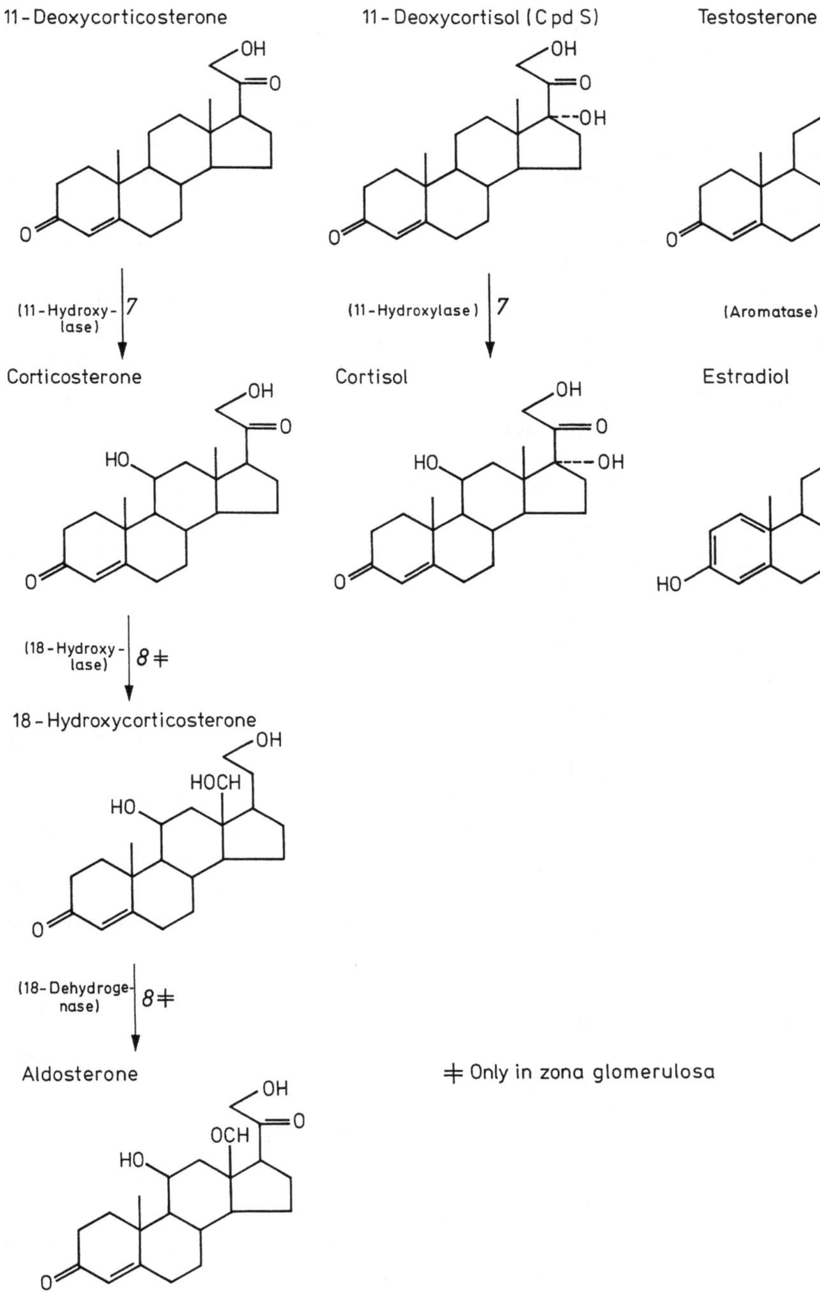


**Fig. 4.1.** Major biosynthetic pathways for adrenal steroids: *1* occurs in lysosomes; *2* transport to mitochondria; *3* hydroxylation and side-chain cleavage (see Fig. 4.2); *4* transport to smooth endoplasmic reticulum (SER); *5a* hydroxylation and *5b* oxidation and isomerization in SER; *6* hydroxylation in SER; *7* mitochondrial hydroxylation; *8* mitochondrial hydroxylation and oxidation

proteins induced by glucocorticoids. In those instances where glucocorticoids induce catabolic effects and eventual cell death (such as in rat thymocytes, which are lysed by glucocorticoids), it is postulated that these events are also initiated by induction of a protein or some other transcriptional event, the nature of which is unknown.

In addition to this "classic" description of the mechanism of glucocorticoid action, there have been suggestions that these hormones may in some instances act on membrane surfaces, perhaps by altering phospholipid composition (Nelson et al. 1979). It has been suggested that the effect of glucocorticoids on stabilizing lysosomal membranes may explain some of the physiological responses to these steroids (Weissmann 1972). However, the hormonal concentrations at which such stabilization is seen are greater than those required for most other glucocorticoid effects. Stabilization of lysosomal membranes, thus preventing release of lysosomal enzymes, may explain the anti-inflammatory actions of steroids in pharmacological doses.

One interesting aspect of the action of corticosteroids is the mechanism by which they exert so-called permissive effects. This signifies that, although the corticosteroids themselves may not induce a given metabolic effect, physiological concentrations of glucocorticoids are necessary for such an effect as mediated by action of other hormones. Examples of permissive effects are those involved in the hormonal regulation of glucose metabolism. Adrenalectomized animals manifest impaired stimulation of gluconeogenesis by either glucagon or epinephrine. This can be corrected by glucocorticoid administration. The defect in the glucocorticoid-deficient animal is the result of an inability of epinephrine to activate phosphorylase, perhaps requiring glucocorticoid-induced alterations in calcium transport, since raising perfusate calcium concentrations also restores activity of phosphorylase b kinase (Miller et al. 1971). Another suggestion is that the glucocorticoid permissive effect is indirectly mediated via enzyme synthesis, since some permissive effects (i.e., on epinephrine-induced lipolysis) are blocked by cycloheximide. It is of interest that the reactions in which glucocorticoids exhibit permissive effects are those in which the hormones that effect the reaction do so via activation of the cAMP system. This suggests that there is increased glucocorticoid-induced synthesis of specific mRNA for substrates on which cAMP acts. There is no evidence that cAMP as such acts as an intracellular "second messenger" to carry out direct cellular effects of glucocorticoids via adenyl cyclase stimulation (Thompson and Lippman 1974).

On an "organismic" level, many of the physiological effects of glucocorticoids involve a redistribution of metabolic energy from lipids, protein, and nucleic acids toward carbohydrates, making the latter a readily available energy reserve. This is accomplished by increased glycogenolysis, increased gluconeogenesis, and decreased tissue glucose uptake (except in brain, red blood cells, and heart), with the excess glucose generated stored as liver glycogen.

At the present time, it is probably not possible to present a unified hypothesis to explain all glucocorticoid actions on varied tissues. It is also not clear that the actions described with regard to inhibition of glucose uptake, stimulation of protein(enzyme) induction, or interrelationship with the cAMP

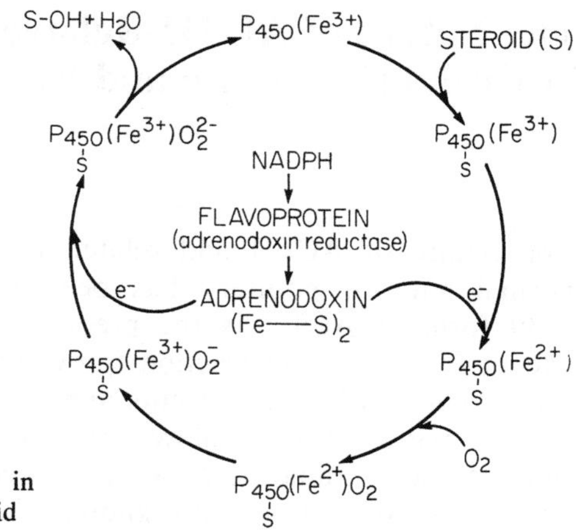


**Fig. 4.2.** Possible enzymatic events involved in steroid hydroxylation in mitochondria. *S*, steroid

system explain all of the observed actions noted in Table 4.1. Although many of the actions are mediated through cytosol receptor proteins and possibly via lysosomal stabilization, the existence of effects that are not explained by the receptor mechanism may indicate other mechanisms of glucocorticoid action. Many effects of corticoids may occur more or less independently of one another in different systems, implying some degree of specificity thus far unexplained. Table 4.1 attempts to list the more commonly accepted actions of glucocorticoids and relate them to the clinical manifestations seen in endogenous Cushing's disease and syndrome and with exogenous corticosteroid administration.

## References


Baxter JD, Forsham PH (1972) Tissue effects of glucocorticoids. Am J Med 53:573–589

Leung K, Munck A (1975) Peripheral actions of glucocorticoids. Ann Rev Physiol 37:245–272

Miller TB, Exton JH, Park CR (1971) A block in epinephrine-induced glycogenolysis in hearts from adrenalectomized rats. J Biol Chem 246:3672–3678

Nelson DH, Ruhmann-Wennhold A, Murray DK (1979) Phospholipid mediation of corticosteroids. Endocrine Soc, 61st Ann Meeting, p 232 (Abstract)

Rousseau GG (1978) Molecular mechanisms of glucocorticoid hormone action and their physiopathological implications. In: James VHT, Serio M, Giusti G, Martini L (eds) The endocrine function of the human adrenal cortex. Academic Press, New York, pp 137–154

Rousseau GG, Baxter JD, Tomkins GM (1972) Glucocorticoid receptors: Relations between steroid binding and biological effects. J Mol Biol 67:99–115

Thompson EB, Lippman ME (1974) Progress in endocrinology and metabolism. Mechanism of action of glucocorticoids. Metabolism 23:159–202

Weissmann G (1972) Lysosomal mechanisms of tissue injury in arthritis. N Engl J Med 286: 141–147

*Chapter 5*

# The Nature of ACTH-Related Peptides in Cushing's Disease and Syndrome

The nature of ACTH and related peptides present in and secreted from normal anterior pituitary has been discussed in Chap. 1. As noted, the 1–39 form of ACTH is the predominant form identified in the pituitary, except for a variable fraction (previously termed big ACTH) eluting in the void volume, which represents approximately 15 %–25 % of the total ACTH content (Gewirtz and Yalow 1974; Orth and Nicholson 1977). Since at the time of these studies the extent of cross-reactivity of available antibodies with pro-opiocortin was not known, the actual amount of precursor present cannot be definitively stated.

It is generally agreed that ACTH and LPH are present in anterior pituitary in equimolar concentrations (Lowry et al. 1977; Liotta et al. 1978). Variable amounts of $\gamma$-LPH have been reported. Scott and Lowry (1974) noted a small amount of acidic material reactive in their $\beta$-MSH assay which appeared to have a composition similar to $\gamma$-LPH, although the predominant molecular species present was identified as $\beta$-LPH, whereas Tanaka et al. (1978) found equal or greater amounts of $\gamma$- than $\beta$-LPH. In recent studies in which 7 fresh normal operative pituitaries were examined, using an N-terminal-directed $\beta$-LPH antibody, immunoreactive $\gamma$-LPH-sized material comprised 10–30% of $\beta$-LPH-sized material (Liotta, Falaschi, and Krieger, unpublished observations). Only a minor amount of $\beta$-endorphin is present in normal human anterior pituitary tissue (Liotta et al. 1978; Suda et al. 1979), which is less than that of r-LPH. Similar findings were obtained (Liotta and Krieger 1980) when pulse-chase experiments were performed on anterior pituitary cells incubated with [$^{35}$S] methionine. These studies (utilizing an ACTH antibody) demonstrated incorporation of label into high molecular weight material, then into a 22-17K form of ACTH, and finally into ACTH$^{1-39}$, while $\beta$-LPH (and not $\beta$-endorphin) was the only form detected during a 4 h chase when employing a $\beta$-endorphin antiserum that cross-reacts on an equimolar basis with $\beta$-LPH. In a 6 h labeling experiment, approximately 6% $\beta$-endorphin was detected on a molar basis.

There have been limited studies of the nature of pituitary ACTH in patients with Cushing's disease. We (Krieger et al. 1976) have reported one case showing a "primary" pituitary tumor. Of the ACTH present, 9% had the reported characteristics of big ACTH, utilizing an antibody that reacted with the precursor form on an equimolar basis. This form, however, had a greater percentage of bioreactivity than previously reported for this molecular species. There were also large amounts of biologically inactive C-terminal fragments and small fragments detected by an N-terminal immunoassay. Similar forms were present in the medium from tumor tissue culture, although the percentage of big ACTH was greater, suggesting increased tumor secretion of the precursor form. Assays for other related peptides were not performed, since these studies were carried out before we were aware that the precursor molecule contained both ACTH and LPH, as well as their component peptides. A study (Suda et al. 1979) with small pituitary tumors obtained by transphenoidal operation in patients with Cushing's disease reports that in the adenomas, in contrast to normal pituitary, specific β-endorphin immunoreactivity constituted 26%–92% of the total immunoreactivity measured by β-endorphin antisera (reacting with β-endorphin and β-LPH on an equimolar basis). Immunoreactive ACTH concentrations in the adenomas were two- to tenfold higher than reported for normal pituitary tissue, whereas in the case reported by Krieger et al. the tumor content was one order of magnitude less. (In the latter case, the tumor mass might be great enough to make the total amount of ACTH available greater than that of the normal pituitary. More recently (Suda et al. 1979), it has been reported that such elevated β-endorphin/β-LPH ratios are present even in the pituitary tissue surrounding the adenoma, in which ACTH and β-endorphin plus β-LPH concentrations were extremely low.

The ACTH concentration present in the pituitary tumor (Krieger et al. 1976) was within the wide range of concentrations reported in tumors of patients with the ectopic ACTH syndrome. These concentrations were 0.0001–60.0 μg/mg, with the majority containing less than 1.0 μg/mg, in contrast to the concentration of 0.4–1.0 μg/mg reported for human anterior pituitary (Ratcliffe et al. 1972; Orth et al. 1973; Gewirtz and Yalow 1974; Rees and Ratcliffe 1974; Harata et al. 1976; Himsworth et al. 1977). A large portion of ACTH immunoreactivity appears to be present as high molecular weight material (Orth et al. 1973; Gewirtz and Yalow 1974; Himsworth et al. 1977). These ectopic tumors are also characterized by the presence of great excesses of both extreme N-terminal and C-terminal immunoreactive material and marked differences in ratios of immunoreactivity/bioreactivity obtained when such C- and N-terminal antibodies are used. In contrast to the identical ratios found in normal pituitary, no matter which antibodies are employed, variable immunoreactive/bioreactive ratios are present in such ectopic tumors even when an antibody reacting with the midportion of the molecule is used (values obtained with such an antibody show the best correlation with those obtained by bioassay). Such dissociation of immunological and biological reactivity may be explained by the high proportion of big ACTH present, which has only a small fraction of the biological activity of $ACTH^{1-39}$. In the case reported by Himsworth et al. (1977), it was noted that during the course of the patient's illness the ACTH secreted became biologically less potent, suggesting alteration in tumor processing with progression of the disease. Additional forms of ACTH may also be present in such tumors. There have been several reports, exemplified by that of Nichols and Gourley (1963), in which bioassayable material with adrenal weight-maintaining capacity was detected in tumors devoid of corticosteroid-releasing capacity.

When discussing the nature of ACTH peptides present in ectopic tumors, it is also of interest to consider the nature of ACTH present in tumors that do not clinically manifest the ACTH syndrome. There is substantial literature reporting significant concentrations of immunoreactive ACTH in carcinomas of the lung in patients who exhibit no clinical evidence of Cushing's syndrome (Yalow 1979; Wolfsen and Odell 1979). In the majority of these instances, the predominant form present was big ACTH (which, as mentioned previously, has little inherent biological activity). There does not appear to be any correlation between the ACTH levels present in such tumors and that present in plasma. This observation, together with the occurrence of false-positive elevations of plasma ACTH concentrations nonspecifically secondary to stress or chronic illness, and the overlap of elevated concentrations between those patients who manifest carcinoma and those at high risk (i.e., patients with chronic pulmonary disease), lessens the efficacy of measurements of plasma ACTH as tumor markers.

As yet, there is no clear picture as to whether LPH alone or β-MSH in addition is present in such ectopic tumors. Harata et al. (1976) demonstrated both LPH and β-MSH in tumor tissues of patients with ectopic ACTH syndrome. There is some question as to whether the presence of β-MSH was an artifact of the extraction method employed. In addition, the biological activity of the LPH material characterized was different from that of pituitary-derived β-LPH. Bertagna et al. (1979) have reported secretion of β-LPH, γ-LPH, and β-endorphin by cells derived from an oat cell carcinoma maintained in culture, although the patients from whom the cells were obtained was not diagnosed as having hypercortisolism. More recently, all of these peptides have been detected in tissues and plasma from patients with the ectopic ACTH syndrome (Pullan et al. 1980; Hashimoto et al. 1980).

Very recently, Nakai et al. (1980) have reported evidence for γ-MSH-like immunoreactivity in ectopic ACTH-producing tumors, and Bertagna et al. (1980) have described the presence of a peptide similar to the $NH_2$-terminal half of the precursor molecule (16K) in extracts of tumors and in plasma obtained from patients with Nelson's syndrome.

## References

Bertagna X, Ferard F, Seurier D, Luton JP, Bricaire H, Main ER, Eipper BE (1980) Evidence for a peptide similar to 16K fragment in man: Its relationship to ACTH. J Clin Endocrinol Metab 51:182–184

Bertagna XY, Nicholson WE, Tanaka K, Mount CD, Sorenson GD, Pettengil OS, Orth DN (1979) Ectopic production of ACTH, lipotropin, and β-endorphin by human cancer cells. Structurally related tumor markers. Recent Results Cancer Res 67:16–25

Gewirtz G, Yalow RS (1974) Ectopic ACTH production in carcinoma of the lung. J Clin Invest 53:1022–1032

Harata Y, Matsukura S, Imura H, Nakamura M, Tanaka A (1976) Size heterogeneity of β-MSH in ectopic ACTH-producing tumors: Presence of β-LPH-like peptide. J Clin Endocrinol Metab 42:33–40

Hashimoto K, Takahara J, Ogawa N, Yunoki S, Ofuji T, Arata A, Kanda S, Terada K (1980) Adrenocorticotropin, β-lipotropin, β-endorphin, and corticotropin-releasing factor-like activity in an adrenocorticotropin-producing nephroblastoma. J Clin Endocrinol Metab 50:461–465

Himsworth RL, Bloomfield GA, Coombes RC, Ellison M, Gilkes JJH, Lowry PJ, Setchell KDR, Slavin G, Rees LH (1977) 'Big ACTH' and calcitonin in an ectopic hormone-secreting tumour of the liver. Clin Endocrinol 7:45–62

Krieger DT, Choi HH, Anderson PJ (1976) The characterization of the ACTH produced by a primary pituitary tumour in a patient with Cushing's disease. Clin Endocrinol 5:455–472

Liotta A, Krieger DT (1980) In vitro biosynthesis and comparative posttranslational processing of immunoreactive precursor corticotropin/β-endorphin by human placental and pituitary cells. Endocrinology (in press)

Liotta AS, Suda T, Krieger DT (1978) β-Lipotropin is the major opioid-like peptide of human pituitary and rat pars distalis: Lack of significant β-endorphin. Proc Nat Acad Sci USA 75:2950–2954

Lowry PJ, Silman RE, Hope J (1977) Structure and biosynthesis of peptides related to corticotropins and β-melanotropins. Ann NY Acad Sci 297:49–62

Nakai Y, Tanaka I, Fukata J, Nakao K, Oki S, Takai S, Imura H (1980) Evidence for gamma-MSH-like immunoreactivity in ectopic ACTH-producing tumors. J Clin Endocrinol Metab 50:1147–1148

Nichols J, Gourley W (1963) Adrenal weight-maintaining corticotropin in carcinoma of the lung. JAMA. 185:68–70

Orth DN, Nicholson WE (1977) Different molecular forms of ACTH. In: Krieger DT, Ganong WF (eds) ACTH and related peptides: Structure regulation and action. Ann NY Acad Sci 297:27–46

Orth DN, Nicholson WE, Mitchell WM, Island DP, Liddle GW (1973) Biological and immunological characterization and physical separation of ACTH and ACTH fragments in the ectopic ACTH syndrome. J Clin Invest 52:1756–1759

Pullan PT, Ratter SJ, McLouglin L, Clement-Jones V, Lowry PJ, Besser SM, Rees LH (1980) Adrenocorticotrophin, lipotrophin and opioid peptides in the ectopic ACTH syndrome. VI International Congress Endocrinology, Melbourne, 761 (Abstract)

Ratcliffe JG, Knight RA, Besser GM, Landon J, Stansfeld AG (1972) Tumor and plasma ACTH concentrations in patients with and without the ectopic ACTH syndrome. Clin Endocrinol 1:27–44

Rees LH, Ratcliffe JG (1974) Ectopic hormone production by non-endocrine tumors. Clin Endocrinol 3:263–302

Scott AP, Lowry PJ (1974) Adrenocorticotropic and melanocyte-stimulating peptides in the human pituitary. Biochem J 139:593–602

Suda T, Abe Y, Demura H, Demura R, Shizume K, Tamahashi N, Sasano N (1979) ACTH, β-LPH and β-endorphin in pituitary adenomas of the patients with Cushing's disease: Activation of β-LPH conversion to β-endorphin. J Clin Endocrinol Metab 49:475–477

Tanaka K, Nicholson WE, Orth DN (1978) The nature of the immunoreactive lipotropins in human plasma and tissue extracts. J Clin Invest 62:94–104

Wolfsen AR, Odell WD (1979) Pro ACTH: Use for early detection of lung cancer. Am J Med 66:765–772

Yalow RS (1979) Big ACTH and bronchogenic carcinoma. Ann Rev Med 30:241–248

*Chapter 6*

# Clinical Manifestations of Cushing's Disease and Cushing's Syndrome

As indicated in Table 1.1 there are several etiologies of hypercorticism. Many clinical manifestations are common to all groups, although there are some that will enable clinical distinctions to be made among the various subgroups. For this reason, greatest emphasis in this chapter will be placed on the pathophysiology of Cushing's disease, since the clinical findings associated with this condition are seen in virtually all other causes of Cushing's syndrome. In addition, consideration will be given to the salient clinical features that distinguish the various subgroups of Cushing's syndrome from each other and from Cushing's disease, as well as consideration of other conditions which may have to be differentiated from hypercortisolism per se.

## A. Cushing's Disease

### I. Pathogenesis

This condition has already been defined as hypercorticism occurring in the absence of adrenal or extrahypophyseal neoplasms. The adrenals may be of normal size or bilateral cortical hyperplasia may be present. The nature of the pituitary pathology and the role of the pituitary in the pathogenesis of this disease have been the subject of considerable speculation over the past 5 decades.

Following the publication of Cushing's classic studies (1932), it was generally believed that Cushing's disease was secondary either to the basophil cell hyperplasia that he had demonstrated, or to an adenoma of the pituitary gland. In the 1940s, attention was focused on the adrenal as the primary source of the pathophysiology present, based on the finding of its hyperresponsiveness to ACTH as seen in such patients. A possible pituitary source was discounted, since plasma ACTH levels, obtained with the relatively insensitive bioassay then available, were normal. It is now known that adrenal hyperresponsiveness to ACTH administration can be attributed to sensitization of this gland by exposure to greater-than-normal amounts of corticotropin. When exogenous ACTH is given, therefore, such a primed gland secretes more corticosteroids. It was also not realized at that time that the presence of normal plasma ACTH concentrations was inappropriate for the elevated plasma cortisol concentrations present in such patients, in whom, if normal feedback mechanisms were operative, plasma ACTH levels should be markedly suppressed. Finally, there was also an inadequate appreciation of the phenomenon of circadian variation of plasma ACTH concentrations, and the absence of such variation in Cushing's disease. Today it is recognized that it is possible for patients with this condition to have "normal" morning plasma ACTH concentrations (when peak concentrations are present in normal subjects), but that the presence of similar levels in the late afternoon and early evening (when the nadir of plasma ACTH concentrations is attained in normal subjects) would be decidedly abnormal.

During this era, there were also suggestions that Cushing's disease might be secondary to abnormalities within the CNS. Heinbecker (1944) described postmortem findings of degranulation and swelling in the paraventricular and supraoptic nuclei in some patients with Cushing's disease. The significance of these findings is questionable, since such pathological changes can also be seen in experimental animals given high doses of corticosteroids. There are also postmortem reports of dilatation of the ventricular system, together with some degree of cortical atrophy, in these patients. Again, whether such changes are causative or secondary to the hypercorticism is questionable. There are several reports of hypercorticism associated with increased intracranial pressure secondary to CNS tumors, with regression of the hypercorticism following tumor removal and alleviation of the increased intracranial pressure. A most significant case, suggestive of a CNS etiology, is that reported by Wolff et al. (1964). In this patient, episodic attacks, manifested by nausea, vomiting, fever, emotional disturbance, and marked weight change, were associated with findings during the attacks of facial plethora, hypertension, abnormal glucose tolerance, elevated plasma ACTH levels, and evidence of adrenal hyperfunction. Neurological examination revealed a normal electroencephalogram and evidence of some cortical atrophy and slight ventricular dilatation.

During the 1950s, consideration of the etiology of Cushing's disease shifted back to the pituitary. This was, in part, secondary to the successful use of pituitary irradiation in the therapy of Cushing's disease, even though it was possible that some of the benefits of irradiation were derived from its effects on the nervous system and not primarily on the pituitary gland. Additional evidence of pituitary pathology in Cushing's disease can be deduced on a clinical basis when there are positive roentgenographic findings in the sellar area. The pituitary may be grossly enlarged at the time of diagnosis (10% of cases) (see Table 1.1), with a radiologically visible tumor present on routine sellar X-ray. In other patients, evidence of a microadenoma may be present when sellar polytomography is performed (reports of abnormal findings vary from 20% to 60% of patients, though in many instances there is no correlation between tomographic and subsequent surgical findings) (MacEalern et al. 1976; Tyrrell et al. 1976; Salassa et al. 1978). In still other patients, there may be no roentgenographic evidence of pituitary pathology.

Further evidence in support of a pituitary etiology has been based on autopsy or surgical findings. Table 6.1 indicates the reported incidence of pathological findings in several series. It is apparent that although pituitary tumors occur in patients without clinical evidence of Cushing's disease, their frequency and the percentage of these that are basophilic are less than encountered in patients with this illness. It is of interest that such basophilic adenomata in normal subjects may be demonstrated immunocytochemically to be composed of corticotrophs, without evidence of increased ACTH se-

**Table 6.1.** Pituitary histology (light microscopy)

| Author | (N) | Tumors (%) |
|---|---|---|
| *Cushing's disease* | | |
| Cushing[a] (1932) | 22 | 64 (all basophilic) |
| Thompson and Eisenhardt[b] (1943) | 48 | 81 (85% of these basophilic) |
| Plotz et al.[b] (1952) | 58 | 60 (45% of these basophilic, 7% ↑ basophils) |
| Burke and Beardwell[c] (1973) | 15 | 52 (45% of these basophilic) |
| Ludecke et al.[d] (1976) | 15 | 73 11 cases: 2 adenoma alone<br>9 adenoma + ACTH cell hyperplasia (mostly nodular)<br>4 cases ACTH cell hyperplasia |
| Carmalt et al.[e] (1977) | 13 | 54 (all basophilic or mixed)<br>23 (focal hyperplasia of basophils) |
| *Normal subjects* | | |
| Sussman[f] (1934) | 260 | 8 (50% of these basophilic) |
| Walters et al.[f] (1934) | 1000 | 20 (20% of these basophilic) |
| Daughaday[f] (1974) | – | 25 (small adenomas or localized nests of cellular proliferation) |
| Carmalt et al.[d] (1977) | 200 | 0 |

[a] Surgical or autopsy findings.
[b] Autopsy findings (no comment as to size).
[c] Autopsy findings or at time of pituitary implant.
[d] Transphenoidal Hypophysectomy (complete), Transphenoidal Hypophysectomy (breast cancer).
[e] Transphenoidal Hypophysectomy (partial).
[f] Autopsy findings.

cretion (Kovacs et al. 1978; Horvath et al. 1980). There have been several reports in patients with Cushing's disease (Saeger 1974, 1977; Garcia et al. 1976; Ludecke et al. 1976; Carmalt et al. 1977) of basophilic hyperplasia alone or in association with basophilic adenoma. In one case, transition of hyperplasia to a mucoid adenoma was demonstrated. This may be similar to the concept of prolactin cell hyperplasia reported in patients with hyperprolactinemia, with or without associated demonstrable adenoma (McKeel and Jacobs 1977; Kovacs et al. 1978, 1979). These observations raise the question, an important one with regard to therapy, as to whether the pituitary findings represent an autonomous process or are secondary to excessive hypothalamic stimulation by the postulated CRF. In the former instance, one would expect cure following surgical removal. In the latter, even after surgical cure is accomplished, continued stimulation might result in recurrence. The results of surgery, which may bear on this question, will be discussed subsequently.

There is also experimental evidence that may support the theory of CNS stimulation of pituitary hyperfunction in certain instances of Cushing's disease. Two of the major abnormalities encountered in patients with this condition, namely, altered circadian periodicity of plasma corticosteroid and ACTH concentrations, as well as resistance to dexamethasone suppression, may well represent abnormalities of CNS regulation of pituitary-adrenal function. The finding especially of altered circadian periodicity of plasma growth hormone and prolactin concentrations and absence of stages 3 and 4 slow-wave sleep in patients with Cushing's disease, and persistence of these abnormalities in such patients in whom laboratory and clinical remission has been induced by pituitary irradiation (Krieger and Glick 1974; Krieger 1978b), further supports a CNS etiology. Even Cushing, at a time when there was no awareness of the concepts of present-day neuroendocrinology, may have realized the possibility of a CNS etiology. As early as 1913, he stated, "We are not blind to the fact that it may lurk in the background particularly in the case of the glandular hyperplasias ... some primary derangement of the nervous system."

### II. Signs and Symptoms

This section will deal with the clinical manifestations common to all forms of hypercorticism. Those more characteristic of the various subgroups comprising the classification of Cushing's syndrome will be subsequently discussed. Table 4.1 has summarized both the physiological and the pharmacological effects of glucocorticoids. Many of the clinical manifestations of Cushing's disease are directly related to such effects, together with additive effects of the adrenal androgens that are hypersecreted in such cases.

Table 6.2 lists the percentage incidence of clinical manifestations in Cushing's disease. This condition occurs more frequently in females of reproductive age, although it has been reported at all ages in both males and females. The presence of obesity, particularly in the facial, nuchal, and truncal areas, while sparing the extremities, is characteristic. Such obesity is usually of a moderate degree. The basis for this characteristic pattern may lie in glucocorticoid effects on both fat and protein metabolism. In animals, "brown fat" is markedly increased in response to cortisone treatment (Aronson et al. 1954). Similar effects in the human may account for the special prominence of fat tissue in the posterior aspect of the neck ("buffalo hump") and in the fat pads of the cheeks, leading to the "moon facies." It should be noted that the decreased lipogenesis mentioned in Table 4.1 refers to cortisol effects only on white fat. The effects of the increased secretion of insulin present in hypercorticoid states will act in an opposite manner to increase lipogenesis. The apparent sparing of the limbs may be secondary to muscle atrophy in such patients, reflecting increased protein catabolism, which may be ameliorated to some extent when androgen hypersecretion is present. The associated muscle weakness may be secondary both to the decrease in muscle mass and to associated hyperkalemia. The ultrastructural changes in muscle are those of pronounced mitochondrial damage, similar to that described in patients with steroid-induced myopathy and in animals treated with corticosteroids. Additional findings are thickening of capillary and sarcolemmal basement membrane (Djaldetti et al. 1977).

The degree of hypertension does not appear to be related to sex, duration of symptoms, or extent of elevation of steroid levels. Such hypertension is usually moderate, with increases in both systolic and diastolic pressure. Patients are prone to the cardiovascular manifestations of hypertension, with

**Table 6.2.** Incidence of signs and symptoms in 450 patients with Cushing's syndrome (Data of Dr. L. J. Soffer)

| Sign or symptom | Incidence (%) |
|---|---|
| Moon facies | 88[a] |
| Obesity | 86[a] |
| Buffalo hump | 54 |
| Weakness | 67 |
| Fatigue | 74 |
| Hypertension | 85 |
| Plethora | 77 |
| Violaceous striae | 60 |
| Easy bruisability | 59 |
| Ecchymoses | 52 |
| Mild polycythemia | 20 |
| Poor wound healing and leg ulcers | 35 |
| Ankle edema | 57 |
| Puffiness of eyes | 26 |
| Osteoporosis | 58 |
| Back pain and bone pain | 54 |
| Pathologic fractures | 38 |
| Kyphosis | 25 |
| Renal calculi | 20 |
| Urinary frequency and nocturia | 32 |
| Polydipsia | 28 |
| Mental changes | 46 |
| Headache | 40 |
| Neurological symptoms | 34 |
| Menstrual disorders | 77[a] |
| Hirsutism (in females) | 73[a] |
| Acne | 54 |
| Exophthalamos | 14 |

[a] Present at onset of disease.

approximately 40 % showing cardiac enlargement and electrocardiographic evidence of myocardial involvement. Congestive failure and cerebrovascular accidents occur less frequently. However, death from cardiovascular disease is one of the most common complications of untreated hypercorticism. The hypertension appears to be due both to enhanced vascular responsiveness to pressor agents and to increased formation of angiotensin, with variable reports of increased plasma renin substrate, plasma renin activity, and plasma renin concentration, indicating that excessive mineralocorticoid production alone cannot account for the increase in arterial pressure (Krakoff et al. 1975; Dalakos et al. 1978). It should be noted that detectable elevations of mineralocorticoids are only reported occasionally in patients with Cushing's disease, and may be more frequently encountered in adrenal tumors in which 11-hydroxylase activity may be diminished.

At the present time, it is not clear whether the atherosclerotic changes present in patients with Cushing's disease are secondary to sustained hypertension or represent an independent defect. There are variable reports as to the incidence of major atherosclerotic changes, with perhaps more of a cor-

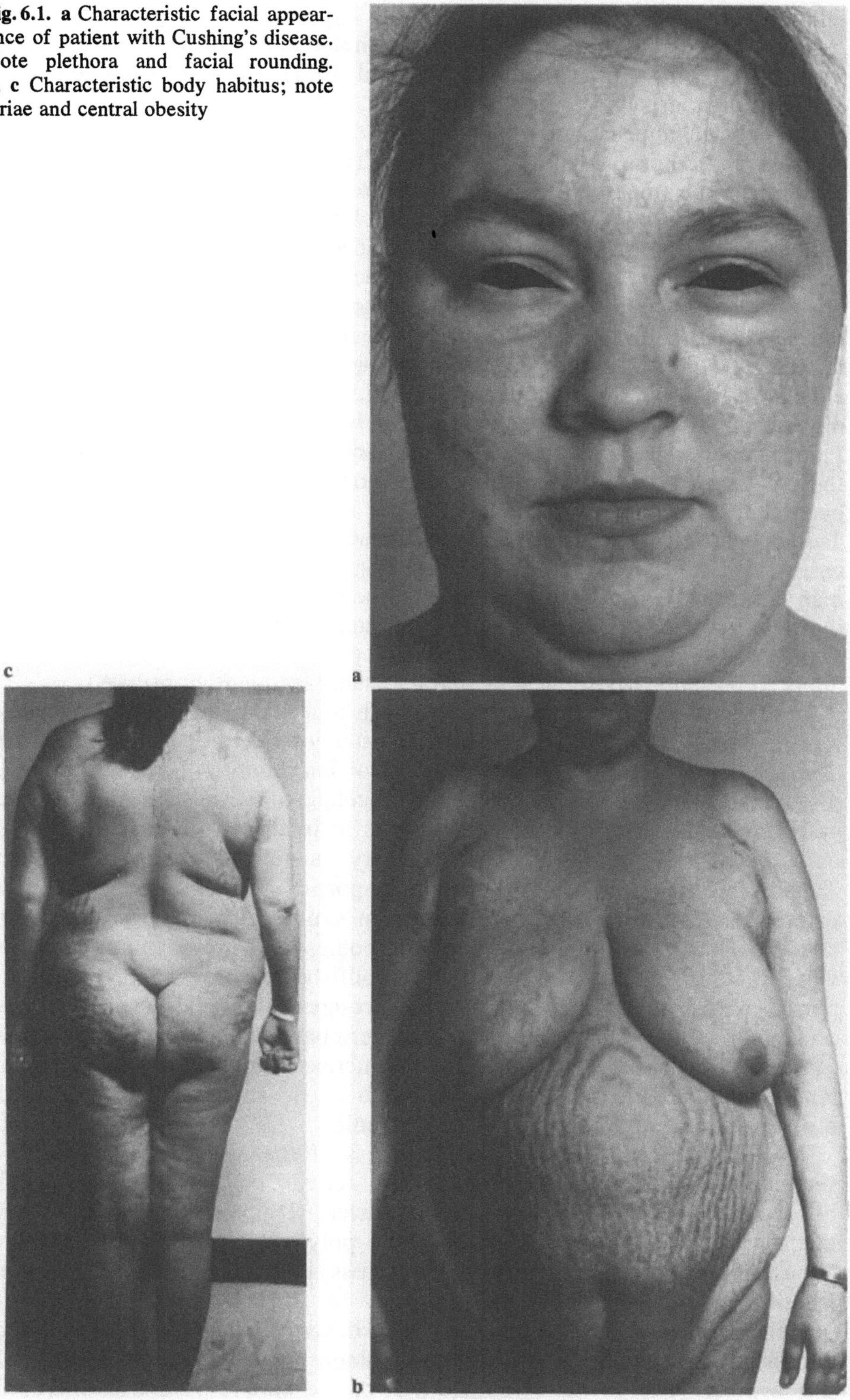

**Fig. 6.1.** **a** Characteristic facial appearance of patient with Cushing's disease. Note plethora and facial rounding. **b, c** Characteristic body habitus; note striae and central obesity

relation with duration of disease than with hypertension. Hypercholesterolemia (not correlated with any changes in metabolic rate) has been noted in approximately 70% of patients (Soffer et al. 1961). There is also a 20% incidence of demonstrated cholelithiasis.

The physical appearance of patients with Cushing's disease is characterized by marked plethora, ecchymoses, thin and fragile skin, and violaceous striae present on the upper portions of the extremities, the breast area, and the abdomen (Fig. 6.1b, c). Plethora may in part be secondary to the polycythemia seen in such patients, which in turn may be secondary to the effect of increased androgen secretion. It should be noted, however, that the plethoric appearance does not necessarily bear a relationship to the hemoglobin content or the red blood cell count. It may in part be due to thinning of the skin secondary to increased catabolism and decreased collagen synthesis, leading to enhanced capillary visibility. This thinning of the skin, associated with increased stretching caused by fat accumulation, has been held to be the basis of the striae. Platelet counts are essentially normal as are the various factors involved in the coagulation process. Paradoxically, shortening of the bleeding time has been reported in animals receiving either acute or chronic hydrocortisone. This is believed to be mediated by decreased prostacyclin generation, which enhances hemostasis by allowing vasoconstriction to be maintained (Blajchman et al. 1979). These data suggest that the hemorrhagic manifestations seen in these patients are probably due to enhanced capillary fragility rather than to any primary hematotologic defect. Similar considerations would apply to the poor wound healing and leg ulcers frequently observed.

Symptoms related to osteoporosis, such as back pain, bone pain, pathological fractures, and kyphosis, are not usually evident at the time of onset of disease, but occur frequently in cases of long duration. The combination of increased catabolism, suppression of collagen synthesis, and decreased gastrointestinal absorption of calcium due to inhibition of 25-hydroxylation of calciferol, as well as increased urinary calcium excretion (as noted in Table 4.1) may all contribute to the osteoporosis. Radiographic evidence of osteoporosis is frequently encountered in skull, extremities, and vertebral column. The weakening of the vertebral bodies leads to bulging of the intervertebral discs, with a characteristic "codfish vertebrae" appearance. Reported symptoms of backache and the presence of kyphosis are often secondary to compression fractures of the vertebral bodies. The hypercalciuria present may also be responsible for the increased incidence of renal calculi noted in these patients. There appears to be no concordance between the presence of osteoporosis and of renal calculi.

Whether the ankle edema and puffiness of the eyes sometimes seen is secondary to increased mineralocorticoid activity or to enhanced transudation from weakened capillary walls is unclear. It is also unclear as to whether the urinary frequency, nocturia, and polydypsia present are related to hypercalciuria or may additionally express the glycosuria seen in these patients.

Mental changes have frequently been described in patients with hypercorticism, and suicide is one of the common causes of death (Starr 1952). The symptomatology may simulate that of the classic psychoses (paranoia, schizophrenia, mania, or depression), although depression is most often described (Cohen 1980). Anxiety, insomnia, and chronic confusion have also been reported. Similar mental changes have been noted in patients receiving exogenous steroid therapy. It has been reported that normalization of plasma cortisol concentrations in patients with Cushing's disease is effective in relieving the depressive symptoms (Jeffcoate et al. 1979). The presence of increased cortisol secretion and other abnormalities of the hypothalamic-pituitary-adrenal axis in patients with depression who do not manifest signs or symptoms of hypercorticism may sometimes pose diagnostic difficulties, as well as being of theoretical importance.

Until more is known about the pathophysiology of behavior, it is difficult to define the biochemical basis of these changes. As noted above, corticosteroids affect enzymes involved in serotonin synthesis, both decreases and increases being reported (Krieger 1978a). Alterations in brain serotonin levels have been implicated in learning and memory processes, as well as in the pathogenesis of several behavioral disorders, including schizophrenia (Essman 1978). Activity of cerebral enzymes, such as glycerol phosphate dehydrogenase and a mitochondrial NADH oxidase, is affected by corticosteroids (Woodbury et al. 1957; Roosevelt et al. 1973). Steroids also alter thresholds of neural excitability and sensory perception. Some of the CNS manifestations noted may be secondary to enhanced levels of ACTH rather than to those of cortisol, in view of the reported findings by de Wied and Gispen (1977) and others of the effects of nonsteroidogenic ACTH fragments on behavior. This possibility appears unlikely, however, since there is no convincing evidence that different psychiatric manifestations are present in patients with Cushing's syndrome secondary to adrenal tumor (with suppressed ACTH levels) than in patients with Cushing's disease (Jeffcoate et al. 1979). It has also been suggested that Cushing's disease may arise as a psychosomatic disorder. Gifford and Gunderson (1970) described what they believe to be a characteristic subset of life experience and personality structure prior to the onset of the symptoms of documented Cushing's disease. In many of these cases, in contrast to Jeffcoate's findings, although remission of the manifestations of hypercorticism occurred after adrenalectomy, psychiatric manifestations persisted over a follow-up period of several years.

Amenorrhea (or oligomenorrhea) is a common finding. As an early manifestation, however, it is present in approximately one-third of patients. Varying degrees of hirsutism are seen, usually confined to moderate body and facial hirsutism, although occasionally clitoromegaly, deepening of the voice, and alopecia are observed. Male patients may show some decrease in libido and body hair. The manifestations in the female are secondary to the direct effect of increased adrenal androgens and their suppressive effects on pituitary gonadotropin secretion. In male subjects, they are secondary to decreased testosterone levels, which may be due to the inhibitory effects of corticosteroids on gonadotropin secretion.

An uncommon manifestation of Cushing's disease (although more common in the ectopic ACTH syndrome) is hyperpigmentation, the basis of which is uncertain. No increase in circulating MSH concentrations has been documented, and $\beta$-lipotropin has only minor pigmentary actions. At present, therefore, the increased levels of ACTH provide the most likely etiology, although there is no correlation between the extent of pigmentation and ACTH concentrations. Increased susceptibility to infection has also been reported. Galactorrhea in the absence of a grossly visible pituitary tumor on X-ray has also been described as an initial symptom, with the other manifestations of Cushing's disease appearing as long as several years afterwards (Young et al. 1967). It should be stressed that not all patients manifest the full-blown clinical picture and that, at times, differentiation, particularly from simple obesity, may pose clinical problems which require laboratory confirmation.

If untreated, Cushing's disease is a progressive malady. Table 6.2 indicates that although the major complications of hypertension, osteoporosis, and mental changes may not be present at the time of onset, they appear with greater frequency over time. Rarely, however, remission (over a 1–5-year follow-up period) occurs without medical or surgical treatment. It should be noted that one of the initial cases described by Cushing (Minnie G.), and observed over a 22-year period, showed signs of spontaneous remission 10 years after the onset of symptoms.

Kammer and Barter (1979) have recently reviewed reported cases of spontaneous remission of hypercorticism: five were in patients with Cushing's disease. In only two of these cases was there adequate laboratory documentation of hypercorticism; two others were diagnosed on the basis of a cushingoid appearance alone. The other case was of interest, in that a cushingoid appearance was present at 18–24 years of age; a spontaneous remission developed with recurrence at age 57, and was documented by laboratory studies. Another recent case is of interest, in that although clinical and laboratory remission appeared to be maintained for approximately 1 year, evidence of some abnormality in the hypothalamic-pituitary-adrenal axis still persisted (Scott et al. 1979). Such spontaneous remissions appear to be in contradistinction to those that represent instances of periodic hormonogenesis, which began to be reported in the decade following Cushing's description. In some instances, the periodic hormonogenesis may be present with no fluctuation or remission in the clinical syndrome. In others, cyclic manifestations of disease may also occur, perhaps dependent on the duration of the period of activity. Periods of hormonal and/or clinical activity could vary from approximately 2 weeks to 2–3 months in duration (the latter instance being seasonal in nature), with symptom-free intervals lasting from several weeks to a year. The usual course is one of increasingly shorter periods of remission over time. More recent cases include those of Wolff et al. (1964) previously cited; cases with shorter cycles of increased hormone production (11–18 days) in association with a carcinoid bronchial adenoma (Bailey 1971; Chajek and Romanoff 1976) and with a chromophobe adenoma (Brown et al. 1973), and a case described by Liberman et al. (1976) in whom laboratory remission appeared to be evident for approximately 30 days of an 86-day cycle. Such spontaneous remission must also be differentiated from those cases in whom remission occurred following adrenal venography (Fellerman et al. 1970; Melby 1972) or following the intramuscular injection of ACTH (Pratt et al. 1974), in which remission was presumably a consequence of infarction of adrenal tissue. There has also been one well-documented and one less well-documented case of remission in patients with Cushing's syndrome secondary to adrenal cortical adenoma (Ovlisen and Andersen 1966; Balu et al. 1975).

## III. Cushing's Disease and Pregnancy

As noted above, infertility in .association with menstrual disturbances is a frequent concomitant of hypercorticism. There have been a number of reports of Cushing's syndrome and pregnancy (Parra and Cruz-Krohn 1966; Kreines and Devaux 1971; Grimes et al. 1973). In four of the cases, unilateral adrenalectomy was performed for adenoma or carcinoma during pregnancy, which then subsequently pursued a normal course. In the remainder of the cases, there was an approximate incidence of abortion, prematurity, and stillbirth of 50%. Where the pregnancy continues, however, there are no data suggesting any possible fetal abnormalities. No somatic malformations have been reported in the fetuses or stillborn infants of such pregnancies, although an overall decrease in adrenal gland weight, with premature involution of the fetal zone and proliferation of the adult zone, has been noted. There has been one report of neonatal adrenal insufficiency as a complication of maternal Cushing's syndrome. This case responded to hydrocortisone and saline infusion (Kreines and Devaux 1971), although in the absence of anatomical data the possibility of a fetal adrenal hemorrhage could not be ruled out.

To date, there are no reports of long-term follow-up of infants born to mothers with active Cushing's disease or syndrome. This is of interest when one considers the experimental observations in rats, that pharmacological amounts of glucocorticoid may affect brain cell division and differentiation (Weichsel 1977). The available data regarding the pharmacological use of cortisone for treatment of other diseases during the course of pregnancy (Bongiovanni and McPadden 1960; Yackel et al. 1966; Herbst 1974: Schatz et al. 1975) report no evidence to suggest an increased incidence of malformations or growth retardation in fetuses of such patients. Apgar scores, which can be used as an index of a CNS effect, show no difference between control groups and infants born to patients receiving short-term glucocorticoid treatment for prevention of the respiratory distress syndrome (Liggins and Howie 1972; Caspi et al. 1976).

## IV. Cushing's Syndrome and Disease in Children

As will subsequently be discussed in greater detail, adrenal tumors (adenomas or carcinomas) account for approximately 80% of the cases in children. It appears that, in children over 7 years of age, hyperplasia may equal or exceed adrenal tumor in frequency. Similar to the sex-related incidence of adrenal hyperplasia, these tumors appear to be more frequent in female subjects. When tumor is present, virilization may dominate the clinical picture. In children with Cushing's disease (McArthur et al. 1972), the clinical manifestations are similar to those reported for the adult, except that obesity is universally reported and shortness of stature is present in 84% of such patients. The cause of such growth suppression is open to some question. It appears that children are less susceptible to suppression of growth hormone secretion following exogenous glucocorticoid administration than are adults. Normal, partial, and complete suppression of growth hormone responses to insulin-induced hypoglycemia have been reported in children with Cushing's syndrome (Stickland et al. 1972).

### V. Familial Cushing's Syndrome

There has been one report of the occurrence of familial Cushing's syndrome in four (two male, two female) of seven siblings, with clinical manifestations appearing around puberty in three of the subjects and onset in the fourth ocurring at approximately 30 years of age. A four-generation genealogical study of both branches of the family revealed no other cases of adrenal hyperfunction. In three of the subjects, adenomatous hyperplasia (see below) was present, while, in the fourth, an uncharacterized tumor was found (Arce et al. 1978).

### VI. Nelson's Syndrome

This clinical condition was originally described (Nelson et al. 1958) in a case of Cushing's disease (in whom the pituitary fossa was initially at the upper limits of normal size on X-ray study) who, 3 years following bilateral adrenalectomy, showed hyperpigmentation, decreased visual acuity, evidence of sellar enlargement and destruction, and marked elevation of plasma ACTH concentrations and urinary MSH activity (Fig. 6.2). It was postulated that the decrease from pathologically elevated plasma corticosteroid concentrations following adrenalectomy served to decrease negative feedback mechanisms, with resultant hypersecretion of ACTH.

With regard to the mechanism of the development of such pituitary tumors, it is of interest that there have been reports of the development of pituitary adenomas with associated ACTH hypersecretion in two patients with Addison's disease. In one patient the duration of disease was 9 years, in the other 28 years. In both patients glucocorticoid replacement therapy may not have been optimal (Himsworth et al. 1978; Jara-Albarran et al. 1979). In one case (Himsworth et al. 1978), after adjustment of medication recalcification of the sella and decrease in sellar size occurred, associated with a decrease in pigmentation. In the other patient, it is interesting to note that, in addition to the markedly elevated ACTH levels present, circadian rhythmicity was absent. Absence of such rhythmicity is characteristic of patients with Cushing's disease or Nelson's syndrome, and is not seen in patients with Addison's disease, who manifest normal circadian rhythmicity of plasma ACTH concentrations.

---

**Fig. 6.2.** Findings in patients with Nelson's disease. **a** Characteristic hyperpigmentation and freckling. Note that hyperpigmentation, although diffuse, is greatest in exposed parts. **b** Hyperpigmentation of mucous membrane ▸

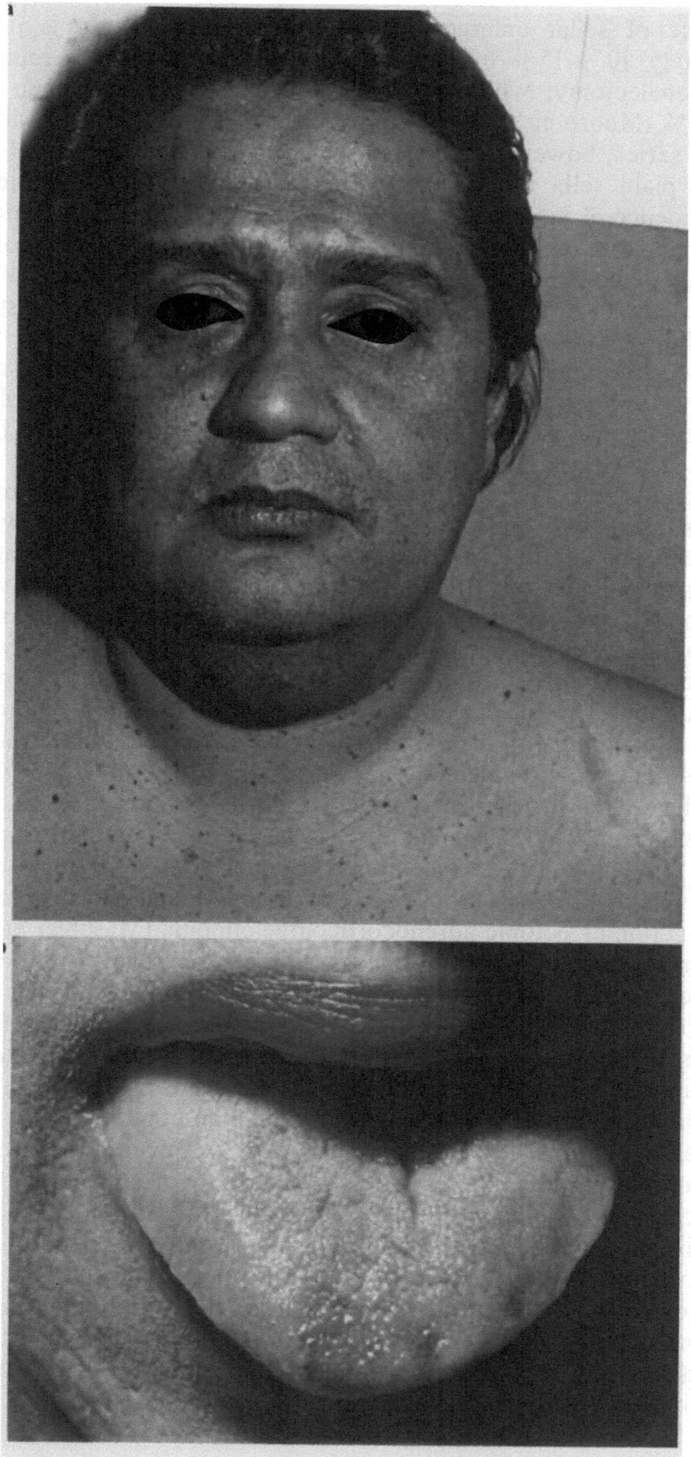

**Fig. 6.2**

Evidence of sellar enlargement on routine sellar X-ray is present in approximately 10%–15% of patients with Cushing's disease following bilateral adrenalectomy, whereas increased pigmentation has been reported in 35%–45% (Moore et al. 1976; Hopwood and Kenny 1977; Nabarro 1977). In another series, however (Weinstein et al. 1976), abnormalities of the sella turcica on plain sella radiographs were noted in 60% of 22 patients who showed evidence of increased pigmentation following bilateral adrenalectomy for Cushing's disease and, in the remaining nine patients, hypocycloidal tomography demonstrated sellar abnormalities (although minimal in size). In children, there is a 25% incidence of pituitary tumors demonstrated on routine sellar X-rays. The frequency of occurrence of associated visual or neurological abnormalities in the presence of pituitary tumor is not clear, but appears to be approximately 25%. Therefore, in a large proportion of patients the sellar enlargement will be asymptomatic and detectable only on follow-up X-rays.

In both adults and children there seems to be an even greater preponderance of female subjects with Nelson's syndrome than is seen in patients with Cushing's disease. The duration of Cushing's disease in patients prior to adrenalectomy does not appear to differ in those patients who subsequently develop evidence of Nelson's syndrome from those who do not. The time of appearance of pituitary enlargement may vary from 6 months to 16 years, but there is no comparable information regarding the time course of appearance of pigmentation. The incidence of development of Nelson's syndrome does not appear to diminish with the use of concomitant pituitary irradiation at the time of bilateral adrenalectomy (Moore et al. 1976; Wild et al. 1973).

Unusual variants have been reported, such as the presence of coexistent Nelson's syndrome and Cushing's disease (secondary to stimulation of adrenal tissue remaining postadrenalectomy) (Bonner et al. 1979) and the appearance of hypercortisolism associated with an abdominal mass, which proved to be a functioning ectopic adrenocorticomyelolipoma (Maschler et al. 1979). In addition to stimulation of adrenal tissue by the high levels of ACTH present in such patients, stimulation of adrenal rests in the gonads has also been reported (Hamwi et al. 1963; Baranetsky et al. 1979; Krieger et al. 1978). Such stimulation had been commonly reported in patients with congenital adrenal hyperplasia, but has not been noted in Nelson's syndrome, save for the three cited reports, the first of which was in a woman and the two others in males. The female patient showed amenorrhea and virilization; laparotomy revealed multiple paraovarian tumors, the microscopic appearance of which closely resembled the morphology of testicular and paratesticular tumors reported in male subjects with this syndrome. In the male patients, presence of tumor was evident on gonadal palpation. In both male subjects there was evidence of cortisol, but not of testosterone production by the tumor. In the case reported by Krieger et al. (1978), serum androgen concentrations were actually decreased, presumably secondary to ACTH effect on suppression of gonadotropin levels.

## VII. Adrenal Pathology

The adrenal glands in Cushing's disease may be normal or increased in size (the weight of a normal adrenal gland is up to 6 g). In the series recorded by Soffer et al. (1961), normal-sized adrenal glands were present in 50 % of the cases, whereas in other series adrenal weights varied from 8.5 to 17.5 g. In approximately 20 % of the patients, multiple and bilateral areas of adenomatous hyperplasia were present rather than simple hyperplasia. These tended to occur in the larger sized adrenal glands, and are different from what has been described (see below) as micronodular hyperplasia. In the series reported by Plotz et al. (1952), adrenal enlargement was present in the majority of cases.

## VIII. Animal Models of Cushing's Disease

To date, Cushing's disease has been reported in two species. In the dog, this condition has been reported in a number of different breeds. Clinical manifestations include polyuria, polydypsia, loss of hair, abdominal enlargement, lethargy, muscle weakness, hyperpigmentation, and occasionally calcinosis cutis. The most frequent pathological finding is bilateral adrenal hyperplasia and, less commonly, neoplasia of the adrenal cortex. Such bilateral hyperplasia is frequently characterized by the appearance of large nodules in the adrenal cortex. There is some question as to the percentage of cases with associated pituitary tumors. In one report (Schechter et al. 1973), tumors of the pars intermedia were present in seven of eight animals on which autopsies were performed. Cases have also been reported in the horse (Moore et al. 1979), also characterized by tumors of the pars intermedia (Pauli et al. 1974) with similar manifestations.

## IX. Variant of Micronodular Hyperplasia

This is an unusual form of Cushing's disease which has been reported mostly in female subjects 2–21 years of age (Ruder et al. 1974). Its onset may precede these ages, in view of the marked extent of osteopenia present when first diagnosed. These patients differ from those with classic adrenal cortical hyperplasia with regard to the nature of the adrenal pathology present and to clinical and laboratory manifestations of the disease. Osteopenia may be the major manifestation, and in some instances may overshadow the mild manifestations of hypercortisolism. In all instances, the adrenals are normal or decreased in weight, and are characterized by the presence, diffuse throughout the gland, of many small nodules containing black or brownish pigment (melanin or lipofuscin). Atrophy of internodular adrenal tissue may be present. Since in many instances plasma ACTH concentrations are low or undetectable, it has been hypothesized that the disease is primarily adrenal in origin (Ruder et al. 1974). An alternative point of view is that this entity may begin with ACTH hypersecretion, with the eventual occurrence of autonomous adrenal function.

These hypotheses may be supported by a recent report (Schteingart and Tsao 1980) of a patient with coexistent pituitary adrenocorticotropin-dependent Cushing's syndrome and a solitary adenoma. In contrast to the usual findings in adrenal adenoma (see below and Chap. 7), this patient was responsive to ACTH; adrenal imaging showed bilateral but asymmetrical uptake of tracer, and there was continued evidence of hypercortisolism following unilateral adrenalectomy. It should be noted, however, that the remaining adrenal tissue present with the adenoma showed no evidence of hyperplastic changes.

## B. Adrenal Tumors

As seen in Table 6.3, there is little to clinically differentiate hypercorticism secondary to adrenal adenomas from that secondary to Cushing's disease, although a greater degree of virilization may be present in the former. Such adenomas are usually small (2.2–4.0 cm, 6–25 g; Soffer et al. 1961).

Virilization is more frequently seen in cases secondary to adrenal carcinoma. It has been stated that the course is longer in patients whose carcinomas produce more androgen than cortisol. In the latter group, defects of 11-hydroxylation have been reported (Lipsett and Wilson 1962), so that tumors may grow to fairly large size before symptoms of cortisol excess are noted (range 4.5 × 4 × 3 cm to 17 × 3 × 11 cm, weight 30–910 g; Soffer et al. 1961). The major symptoms in cases of carcinoma (Lipsett et al. 1963) are those of abdominal pain, weakness, and weight loss. The most common signs are abdominal mass, distant lymphadenopathy, organomegaly, and leg edema. In 50% of patients there are no symptoms, signs, or laboratory evidence of endocrine activity. Such nonfunctioning tumors are more evident in the 6th decade of life, with a slight preponderance in male subjects, whereas

**Table 6.3.** Clinical features as to differential diagnosis

| | Adrenal adenoma | Adrenal carcinoma | Bilateral hyperplasia | Ectopic tumor | 1° Pituitary tumor |
|---|---|---|---|---|---|
| Clinical course | Slow | Rapid | Slow | Rapid | Slow |
| Clinical manifestations | Mild to moderate | Florid, severe | Mild to moderate | Atypical (i.e., myopathy) | Mild to severe |
| Virilization (♀) or feminization (♂) | Rare | Frequent | Rare | 0 | Rare |
| Palpable suprarenal mass | 0 | + | 0 | 0 | 0 |
| Visual, CNS symptoms | 0 | 0 | 0 | 0 | + |
| Sex of patient | 80% (♀), 20% (♂) | | 80% (♀), 20% (♂)[a] | ♂ > ♀ | |
| Age of patient (majority of cases) | All ages | Comprises 60% of cases in children | 20–40 years | 40–60 years | 20–70 years |
| Pigmentation | 0 | 0 | Rare | Present | Present |

[a] Of adult males with Cushing's disease, however, 90% have hyperplasia.

functioning tumors are more common in the 4th to 6th decade, with a marked predominance in female subjects. When endocrine symptoms are present in women, these consist most frequently (50% of patients) of a combination of hypercorticism and virilization. Virilization alone is the next most common manifestation, while only a small percentage of patients show evidence of hypercorticism alone. In male subjects, evidence of hypercorticism may be present with or without feminization, such as gynecomastia and decreased libido. The median time between the onset of symptoms and diagnosis has been reported to be 8.3 months (Lipsett et al. 1963; Hutter and Kayhoe 1966; Hajjar et al. 1974), with no distinction being made between functioning and nonfunctioning tumors.

Metastases are most frequent locally and to adjacent structures, such as the peritoneum and regional lymph nodes. The most common sites of distant metastases are lung and liver, and, to a lesser extent, distant lymph nodes (53%, 44%, and 11% respectively). Metastases to bone and brain are extremely rare. There are no reports which indicate how frequently, with modern diagnostic techniques, lung and hepatic metastases have been detected at the time of initial presentation, which could considerably modify the therapeutic approach. Without such information it is difficult to know which cases may be potentially resectable at the time of abdominal exploration. Lipsett et al. (1963) reported that in only 18 of 38 patients was it possible to attempt definitive therapy. This report does not state how many displayed some evidence of local extension or blood vessel invasion.

## C. "Primary" Pituitary Tumor

Approximately 10% of patients with Cushing's disease may have a grossly visible pituitary tumor on routine X-ray of the sella turcica prior to any therapeutic intervention. Histologically (tissue obtained at surgery or autopsy), most of these have been described as being chromophobe adenomas (some are mixed, i.e., chromophobe and basophil). Newer methods of immunocytochemistry may well reveal that all of these tumors will exhibit positive immunostaining for ACTH, although such immunostaining can occur in the absence of any clinical symptoms (Horvath and Kovacs 1978). Approximately one-quarter of these tumors have been classified as malignant, as evidenced by local invasiveness or, more rarely, by extracranial metastases (Rovit and Berry 1965). It is of interest that when all cases of documented pituitary carcinoma are considered (Querizo et al. 1975), clinical evidence of hypercorticism is present in one-half of those reported as having blood-borne metastases. One reported case of carcinoma is of special interest (Sheldon et al. 1954), in that evidence of hypercorticism was present in a case of basophil carcinoma with hepatic metastases, in whom no evidence of sellar enlargement was present. In another recently reported case of pituitary carcinoma associated with Cushing's syndrome, routine skull films were normal, while polytomography revealed sellar erosion (Fachnie et al. 1980).

Since the frequency of occurrence of small basophilic adenomas in patients with Cushing's disease is now well recognized, the question arises as to whether those cases with macroscopic adenomata represent a different clinical entity from those of microadenomata or whether they represent a continuum. Similar questions occur in attempting to relate large prolactin-secreting "chromophobe" adenomas to the smaller "prolactinomas" seen only on sellar tomography. The development of macroscopic pituitary tumors in 15 %–20 % of patients with Cushing's disease following adrenalectomy (see below) may point to the existence of a continuum. However, the nature of the clinical symptomatology and the course in patients with macroscopic tumors may be sufficiently different as to warrant special consideration.

In some instances (approximately 25 % of patients), evidence of visual and neurological symptoms (diplopia, visual field defects, blurred vision, oculomotor defects, headache, or attacks of unconsciousness) may precede evidence of Cushing's disease. In others, visual, neurological, and endocrine manifestations may be present simultaneously. More rarely, manifestations of Cushing's disease are present, with an initial course indistinguishable from that associated with small adenomata, but with subsequent development of visual or neurological symptoms. Associated hyperpigmentation occurs more frequently than in "uncomplicated" Cushing's disease. This may be secondary to the more markedly elevated plasma ACTH concentrations present in these patients.

There is general agreement that the pituitary tumors considered under the present heading are more aggressive than those associated with "nonendocrine" disease, i.e., chromophobe adenomas (although of course it is now realized that the latter, for the most part, represent prolactin-secreting adenomas). As indicated in Table 6.4, a higher incidence of extraocular palsy, pituitary apoplexy, metastases, and local invasiveness is seen in pituitary tumors associated with Cushing's disease, indicative of a greater degree of cellular dedifferentiation of these tumors (Rovit and Duane 1969).

**Table 6.4.** Findings in pituitary tumors

| | Cushing's disease | Nonendocrine |
|---|---|---|
| Extraocular palsy | 25% | 5–10% |
| Pituitary apoplexy | 11% | <2% |
| Local invasion | 25% | 5–10% |
| Extracranial metastases | 12% | ? |
| "Malignant" histology | 24% | 10%? |

## D. Ectopic ACTH Production

Following the description of Cushing's syndrome by Harvey Cushing, it became apparent that the clinical manifestations could be associated with tumors of various organs. Originally, such tumors were classified into two groups. The first included endocrine tumors, such as basophil adenomas of the pituitary, adrenal cortical tumors, and perhaps some ovarian tumors. A second group included bronchial carcinomas, other intrathoracic neoplasms (mostly thymomas), and carcinoma of the pancreas. It was soon realized that the association of this latter group of tumors was not fortuitous, but for some time no clear explanation was evident.

The first description of Cushing's syndrome associated with a bronchial carcinoma was apparently reported by Brown (1928). It is of interest that Crooke (1946), who described the hyaline changes in the basophil cells of the anterior pituitary lobe common to all forms of hypercorticism, reported on such changes associated with a tumor of the pancreas. During the 1950s and early 1960s, there were several references to the occurrence of adrenal cortical hyperplasia, with or without clinical manifestations of hypercorticism, in subjects with bronchogenic carcinoma, as well as reports of excessive elevation of plasma corticoids following ACTH infusion in such patients. The significance of such hormonal changes in patients without evidence of clinical hypercorticism will be subsequently discussed. In 1960, Levine and Smith suggested that Cushing's syndrome associated with such tumors might be a consequence of tumor elaboration of corticotropin-like hormone. Confirmation of this was forthcoming within the next year in three reports (Holub and Katz 1961; Meador et al. 1962; Nichols et al. 1962), and was elegantly studied and summarized by Liddle et al. (1969).

Table 6.5 lists criteria for establishing ectopic hormone production. All of these, save for the last, have been satisfied with regard to ectopic ACTH production. Table 6.6 lists the tumors associated with the ectopic ACTH syndrome. It can be seen that those comprising the majority of cases were in the locations cited above in the early reports. A possible basis for production of ACTH by such disparate tissues may come from the APUD concept proposed by Pearse in 1966 and later modified (1977). This describes a group of cells derived from neural tissue (neural tube, neural crest, and the placodes) distributed centrally within the hypothalamus, pineal, and pituitary gland, and peripherally in many tissues (thyroid, melanoblast, adrenal medulla, pancreas, stomach, intestine, lung, urogenital area). Such cells have the capability both of peptide synthesis and of amine precursor uptake and decarboxylation

**Table 6.5.** Criteria for ectopic hormone production

| |
|---|
| Association of tumor with clinical endocrine syndrome, elevated or inappropriate hormone levels |
| Fall in circulating hormone levels and/or regression of clinical manifestations of hormone excess following tumor removal |
| Lack of fall of hormone level if normal gland of origin is removed |
| Arterio-venous hormone gradient across tumor bed |
| Demonstration of hormone in tumor tissue |
| Chemical |
| Immunocytochemical |
| Electron microscopy: secretory granules |
| In vitro secretion |
| Synthesis by tissue |

**Table 6.6.** Tumors associated with ectopic ACTH production

| | Frequency (%) |
|---|---|
| Bronchogenic carcinoma (small cell) | 50 |
| Thymic carcinoma | 10 |
| Pancreatic carcinoma (islet cell) (carcinoid) | 10 |
| Thyroid carcinoma (medullary) | 5 |
| Bronchial adenoma (carcinoid type) | 5 |
| Pheochromocytoma, neuroblastoma | 5 |
| Others (parotid, breast, gall bladder, colon, testis, ovary, prostate, uterus, kidney, liver, esophagus, trachea, gut carcinoid, cervix, argentaffinoma) | 15 |

(APUD). The function of these cells as a "third" neural system is still being explored. When tumors of such cells arise, evidence of ectopic peptide hormone production may be seen.

The clinical manifestations of the ectopic ACTH syndrome may vary. This is in part dependent on the biological nature of the tumor, i.e., whether it is rapidly or slowly growing. In the case of rapidly growing tumors (such as those of the lung), the clinical course may be dominated by symptoms of the primary disease as well as by weakness, muscle wasting, extreme myopathy, diabetes mellitus, hypertension, and hypokalemic alkalosis. Hyperpigmentation may also be present. Its presence and that of hypokalemia may be the only clues to tumor production of ACTH. The pathogenesis of the hypokalemia is uncertain; it has been ascribed to excessive desoxycorticosterone and corticosterone secretion. The hyperpigmentation may be secondary both to the elevated ACTH concentrations present and perhaps to actual secretion of $\beta$-MSH by the tumor.

The characteristic clinical manifestations of Cushing's syndrome do not develop in these patients, probably because of the relatively short duration of exposure to elevated corticosteroid concentrations. In addition, such tumors may secrete forms of ACTH which are less biologically active than $ACTH^{1-39}$. Survival in the absence of any attempt to correct the adrenal hypersecretion is usually only several months. In contrast to the course just described for rapidly growing tumors, when the ectopic source of ACTH is derived from any of the other tumors noted in Table 6.6, the course may be longer and more similar to that of pituitary Cushing's disease.

Men and women appear to be equally affected, with an age distribution closer to that of classical Cushing's disease, although a significant percentage of cases is reported in the 5th and 6th decades. Evidence of hypercortisolism can precede detection of the underlying tumor, which may first be noted either following unsuccessful treatment by adrenalectomy (Flint and Jacobs 1974) or at autopsy (Mason et al. 1972). Mason has noted that in 26 cases of the syndrome associated with bronchial adenoma, only in ten was the tumor seen radiologically during the first 6 months following the diagnosis of hypercorticism. In eight cases there was at least a year's delay between the diagnosis of Cushing's syndrome and development of radiological evidence of the bronchial tumor, while in seven others the tumor was identified only post mortem. Similar findings have been reported with regard to medullary carcinoma of the thyroid. In three of six patients presenting typical Cushing's syndrome, the diagnosis of medullary carcinoma was established only at autopsy, whereas in patients who also presented hypokalemic alkalosis, the carcinoma was diagnosed before or concomitant with the hypercorticism. One recent case report (Rosenberg et al. 1978) noted severe osteopenia as a principal manifestation.

Although in some instances, as noted, the clinical course associated with this second group of tumors may be relatively indolent (Morse et al. 1967), in many the presence of hypokalemic alkalosis, peripheral edema, and a more rapidly progressive course of the disease than is usually seen with pituitary ACTH excess may lead to suspicion of ectopic corticotropin production. Occasionally (see below), laboratory tests may aid in differentiation from classical Cushing's disease, although in a number of instances, as will be noted subsequently, similar responses to testing may be obtained in pituitary-dependent Cushing's disease and in ectopic ACTH production. Sometimes a clue as to etiology may be obtained from histological examination of the adrenals, removed in cases where the diagnosis of ectopic tumor had not been entertained. It has been reported that in bilateral adrenal hyperplasia occurring with pituitary ACTH excess, the zona fasciculata has a wide zone of clear lipid-rich cells, in addition to hyperplasia of the compact cells, while in hyperplasia associated with ACTH-producing tumors other than those of the pituitary, this zone is composed solely of granular compact cells (Mason et al. 1972).

Some of these tumors may also exhibit cyclical secretion of corticotropin, although this mechanism is not understood. There have been case reports of intermittent secretion by carcinoid tumors, both of the lung (Chajek and Romanoff 1976) and thymus (Thorner et al. 1979), as well as in pheochromocytoma (Rees et al. 1974; Spark et al. 1979). In the case reported by Spark, there were simultaneous fluctuations of urinary catecholamine and plasma ACTH concentrations. In the case reported by Chajek, the cyclic secretion of corticosterone was also associated with cyclic clinical manifestations.

Some symptoms may be related to ectopic production by the tumor of more than one hormone. Originally, tumor production of $\beta$-MSH, $\beta$-LPH, and CLIP was reported. With the realization that these peptides probably all derive from tumor production of the common precursor molecule pro-opiocortin, it is no longer tenable to consider such citations as evidence of tumor production of multiple hormones. Cases have, however, been reported (Table 6.7) of tumor production of vasopressin, oxytocin, and occasionally of neurophysin. In some of the cases cited this was presumptive, based on determination of serum and urine osmolalities, while in others, peptides were quantified by radioimmunoassay and/or bioassay. The presence of vasopressin

**Table 6.7.** Other hormones produced by ACTH-secreting tumors

| Tumor | Hormone | Reference |
|---|---|---|
| Oat cell cancer, lung | AVP[a] | O'Neal et al. (1968)<br>Cullen and Tomlinson (1968)<br>Hirata et al. (1976)<br>Coscia et al. (1977) |
| Bronchial carcinoid | AVP, neurophysin | Bailey (1971) |
| Oat cell cancer, lung | AVP, oxytocin, neurophysin, prolactin, insulin | Rees et al. (1974) |
| Oat cell cancer, lung | CRF | Upton and Amatruda (1971) |
| Pancreatic islet cell | | Yamamoto et al. (1976) |
| Colon cancer | CRF | Suda et al. (1977) |
| Medullary cancer, thyroid | CRF, PRF | Birkenhager et al. (1976) |
| Hepatic cancer (?) | Calcitonin | Himsworth et al. (1977) |
| Pancreatic islet cell | Gastrin | Law et al. (1965) |

[a] Arginine vasopressin

may explain the inability of patients with the ectopic ACTH syndrome to clear a water load. This has generally been attributed to the effect of hypokalemia on the renal concentrating mechanism, but may in fact be due to excessive vasopressin production. It is also intriguing that, in several instances, a given tumor has been shown to produce ACTH and material with CRF-like activity which has been demonstrated to be different from vasopressin. Finally, in keeping with the APUD concept, oat cell lung carcinomas (noncarcinoid) contain ACTH and serotonin (Mosonyi et al. 1971; Horai et al. 1973). The cases reported by Mosonyi et al. may also have secreted catecholamines. Since the oat cell carcinoma is suggested to be a malignant variant of the bronchial carcinoid tumor (it is derived from the bronchial Kultschitzky-type cell belonging to the APUD cell series), the presence of serotonin and ACTH in the oat cell carcinoma would appear to be derived from the potential capacity of the ancestor cells from which the tumor arises.

## E. Differential Diagnosis of Cushing's Disease and Syndrome

Although differential diagnosis is usually made on the basis of laboratory testing (see Chap. 7), certain clinical features may be helpful. There are two types of differential diagnosis to be considered. The first is the exclusion of conditions which may clinically suggest hypercorticism (but with normal endocrine function), as well as instances in which clinical and/or laboratory evidence of hypercorticism may be present, but which, on the basis of present knowledge, do not represent actual endocrine disease. Cases of obesity, depression, and alcoholism fall into this category. The other type of differential diagnosis involves elucidation of the cause of established hypercorticism. The salient features of such differential diagnosis are indicated in Table 6.3. It can be seen that a clinical distinction between hypercorticism secondary to an adrenal adenoma and secondary to pituitary-dependent

Cushing's disease is difficult. Adrenal carcinoma may be suspected by age of onset, the rapidity of the course, and the frequent association of symptoms of virilization or feminization indicative of hormone secretion other than cortisol by the neoplastic tissue. In cases of ectopic ACTH secretion, the typical clinical manifestations (rapid course, the association of hyperpigmentation, and age of onset) are clues to diagnosis, while the presence of associated visual symptomatology and hyperpigmentation in a case of manifest hypercorticism would point to a primary pituitary tumor.

When considering "nonendocrine" syndromes which may simulate hypercorticism, the situation most frequently encountered is that of obesity (Table 8). Hypertension and menstrual disturbances may also be present in such patients. Differential diagnosis is usually based on laboratory testing. However, the extent of weight increase is usually greater in patients with simple obesity than in those with Cushing's syndrome, in whom the obesity may be more apparent (i.e., secondary to altered distribution of body fat) than real. Obesity is also more generalized in simple obesity, in contrast to the truncal obesity characteristic of states of hypercorticism (except in the ectopic syndrome, which may not manifest such a change). The striae present in simple obesity are usually pink, and shorter and narrower than the purplish striae in hypercorticism, since in the obese subject the striae reflect the thinning and stretching of skin by fat accumulation, thus rendering the underlying vessels visible, whereas in patients with hypercorticism they reflect additional associated defects in capillary fragility and the presence of polycythemia.

Mention has already been made of the frequency of mental changes in patients with Cushing's syndrome. As will be noted in the sections on laboratory diagnosis, depressed patients share many of the endocrine abnormalities seen in patients with Cushing's disease. Such depressed patients have none of the clinical stigmata of hypercorticism, unless obesity is present as an incidental finding. Of interest is the possible relationship between the mental alterations seen in patients with true Cushing's disease and the altered laboratory findings, suggestive of hypothalamic-pituitary-adrenal dysfunction, present in patients with depression. Recently, there has been much interest in altered neurotransmitter metabolism in various categories of psychiatric disease. The interrelationships among postulated neurotransmitter abnormal-

**Table 6.8.** Differential diagnosis of obesity and Cushing's syndrome

| | Obesity | Cushing's syndrome |
|---|---|---|
| Body weight increase | ++ | + |
| Nature of obesity | General | Truncal |
| Striae | Pink, short, narrow | Violaceous, long, wide |
| Cortisol secretory rate | Normal, + | + |
| Urinary 17-OHCS | Normal, + | ++ |
| Urinary free cortisol | Normal | + |
| Plasma 17-OHCS | Normal | Elevated |
| Circadian variation | Present | Absent |
| Dexamethasone suppression (2 mg/day for 2 days) | Suppression | No suppression |

ities, psychiatric disease, and endocrine disturbances are still unclear. The first major question is whether the two latter variables are both sequellae of a common neurotransmitter disturbance or whether the altered behavior present in psychiatric disease is in itself directly responsible for production of endocrine changes. The suggestion has been made (Gifford and Gunderson 1970) that Cushing's disease may be a psychophysiological response to bereavement, or the emotional equivalent, in predisposed individuals with disturbed hypothalamic-pituitary regulation of adrenal activity. Other endocrine abnormalities have been reported in patients with depression, such as the presence of plasma growth hormone or gonadotropin responses to TRH, and occasionally prolactin responsiveness to luteinizing hormone-releasing factor (LHRF) (Brambilla et al. 1978). An additional problem, the answer to which may provide some insights into the pathophysiology of hypercorticism, concerns the question as to why depressed patients with laboratory evidence of hypercorticism do not show any of its common clinical manifestations.

There have been several recent reports of alcohol-induced pseudo-Cushing's syndrome (Smals et al. 1976; Frajria and Angeli 1977; Rees et al. 1978; Lamberts et al. 1979). Of the 11 reported cases, four were female subjects (age range 30–56 years). All patients presented a cushingoid appearance with characteristic obesity, plethora, and striae. Several cases were noted to have associated hypertension. In three, parotid enlargement was noted, and not specifically commented upon in the other cases. All subjects gave a history of alcohol ingestion (varying from 4 liters of gin per week to 6–12 pints of beer daily). Laboratory studies revealed evidence of elevated corticosteroid levels, as determined in plasma, urine, or by measurement of the cortisol secretory rate. In six of eight cases, an abnormal response to 1 mg dexamethasone was reported (see Chap. 7). In two patients in whom such tests were performed, there was also an abnormal response to the administration of dexamethasone (2 mg daily × 2). Comment is made concerning diminished or absent circadian periodicity of plasma corticosteroid concentrations, but in most instances the frequency of plasma steroid level determination is not given, making the validity of this observation difficult to judge. It should be noted, however, that a diminished or absent circadian periodicity of plasma corticosteroid concentrations has been reported in patients with chronic liver disease (Tucci et al. 1966), and all of the alcoholic patients had abnormalities of hepatic function. Progressive impairment in hepatic degradation of cortisol and its resultant decreased clearance could lead to such lessened circadian variation. In all instances, when such patients were hospitalized with discontinuance of alcohol ingestion, the laboratory abnormalities disappeared within several weeks, as did the manifestations of hypercortisolism: It is not stated how long these patients had shown cushingoid appearance.

The basis for hypercorticism under this condition is still not fully understood. Both animal and human experiments (Jenkins and Connolly 1968; Ylikahri et al. 1978) have demonstrated that acute ethanol administration (either intravenously or orally) is associated with elevation of plasma cortisol concentrations. In the latter study, no effect on basal levels of other pituitary trophic hormones, $T_4$, $T_3$, or testosterone was noted, but there was an altered prolactin response to thyrotropin-releasing hormone (TRH), suggesting some alteration of hypothalamic dopaminergic activity. In both animal and human studies, no rise in plasma cortisol concentrations was seen following ethanol administration to hypophysectomized animals or to two subjects with pituitary lesions who also manifested normal responses to vasopressin and decreased responses to pyrogen administration, suggesting pituitary mediation of such a cortisol response. Another possible etiology for hypercorticism has been suggested by observations that corticosteroid-binding globulin was noted to be decreased in two patients (Frajria and Angeli 1977), essentially increasing the amount of free cortisol available. This, however, does not explain the abnormal dexamethasone suppression reported, although it should be noted that there are no reports with regard to whether adequate plasma dexamethasone concentrations have been obtained in the studies of alcoholic patients. A recent report (Cobb et al. 1979) has suggested that in vitro ethanol and acetaldehyde are capable of enhancing rat adrenal corticosterone secretion. Finally, most animal experiments have suggested that the effects of alcohol on the CNS may be due to changes in the concentrations and/or metabolism of brain biogenic amines (Karoum et al. 1970; Hunt and Majchrowicz 1974; Lahti 1975). In view of the known role of these amines in regulation of ACTH secretion, one possibility is that changes in pituitary-adrenal function reflect alteration in central nervous system concentrations of biogenic amines.

## References


Arce B, Licea M, Hung S, Padron R (1978) Familial Cushing's syndrome. Acta Endocrinol 87:139–147

Aronson SM, Teodorn CV, Adler M, Schwartzman G (1954) Influence of cortisone upon brown fat of hamsters and mice. Proc Soc Exp Biol Med 84:214–218

Bailey RE (1971) Periodic hormonogenesis: A new phenomenon. Periodicity in function of a hormone-producing tumor in man. J Clin Endocrinol Metab 32:317–327

Baranetsky NG, Zipser RD, Goebelsmann U, Kurman RJ, March CM, Morimoto I, Stancyzk FZ (1979) Adrenocorticotropin-dependent virilizing paraovarian tumors in Nelson's sydrome. J Clin Endocrinol Metab 49:381–386

Birkenhager MC, Upton GV, Seldenrath HJ, Krieger DT, Tashjian AH (1976) Medullary thyroid carcinoma: Ectopic production of peptides with ACTH-like, corticotropin-releasing factor-like and prolactin production-stimulating activities. Acta Endocrinol 83:280–202

Blajchman MA, Senyl AF, Hirsh J, Surya Y, Buchanan M (1979) Shortening of the bleeding time in rabbits by hydrocortisone caused by inhibition of prostacyclin generation by the vessel wall. J Clin Invest 63:1026–1035

Blau N, Miller WE, Miller ER, Cervi-Skinner SJ (1975) Spontaneous remission of Cushing's syndrome in a patient with an adrenal adenoma. J Clin Endocrinol Metab 40:659–663

Bongiovanni AM, McPadden AJ (1960) Steroids during pregnancy and possible fetal consequences. Fertil Steril 11:181–186

Bonner RA, Mukai K, Oppenheimer JH (1979) Two unusual variants of Nelson's syndrome. J Clin Endocrinol Metab 49:23–29

Brambilla F, Smeraldi E, Sacchetti E, Negri F, Cocchi D, Muller EE (1978) Deranged anterior pituitary responsiveness to hypothalamic hormones in depressed patients. Arch Gen Psychiatry 35:1231–1238

Brown RD, VanLoon GR, Orth DN, Liddle GW (1973) Cushing's disease with periodic hormonogenesis: One explanation for paradoxical response to dexamethasone. J Clin Endocrinol Metab 36:445–451

Brown WHL (1928) A case of pluriglandular syndrome: "Diabetes of bearded women." Lancet II:1022–1023

Burke CW, Beardwell CG (1973) Cushing's syndrome. Quart J Med 42:175–204

Carmalt MHB, Dalton GA, Fletcher RF, Smith WT (1977) The treatment of Cushing's disease by trans-sphenoidal hypophysectomy. Quart J Med 46:119–134

Caspi E, Schreyer P, Weinraub Z, Reif F, Levi L, Mundel G (1976) Prevention of the respiratory distress syndrome in premature infants by antepartum glucocorticoid therapy. Br J Obstet Gynecol 83:187–193

Chajek T, Romanoff H (1976) Cushing's syndrome with cyclical edema and periodic secretion of corticosteroids. Arch Intern Med 136:441–443

Cobb CG, VanThiel DH, Ennis MF, Gavaler JS, Lester R (1979) Pseudocushing's in alcoholics: A mechanism. Clin Res 27:448A (Abstract)

Cohen SI (1980) Cushing's syndrome: A psychiatric study of 29 patients. Br J Psychiatry 136:120–124

Coscia M, Brown RD, Miller M, Tanaka K, Nicholson WE, Parks KR, Orth DN (1977) Ectopic production of antidiuretic hormone (ADH), adrenocorticotrophic hormone (ACTH) and beta-melanocyte-stimulating hormone ($\beta$-MSH) by an oat cell carcinoma of the lung. Am J Med 62:303–307

Crooke AC (1946) Basophilism and carcinoma of the pancreas. J Pathol 58:667–673

Cullen DR, Tomlinson BE (1968) Carcinoma with multiple ectopic hormone secretion and associated myopathy. Postgrad Med J 44:472–476

Cushing H (1913) Psychic disturbances associated with the ductless glands. Am J Insanity 69:965–971

Cushing J (1932) The basophil adenomas of the pituitary body and their clinical manifestations. Bull Johns Hopkins Hosp 50:137–195

Dalakos ThG, Elias AN, Anderson GH Jr, Streeten DHP, Schroeder ET (1978) Evidence for an angiotensinogenic mechanism of the hypertension of Cushing's syndrome. J Clin Endocrinol Metab 46:114–118

Daughaday WH (1974) The adenohypophysis. In: Williams RH (ed) Textbook of endocrinology, 5th ed. Saunders, Philadelphia, pp 31–77

Djaldetti M, Gafter U, Fishman P (1977) Ultrastructural observations in myopathy complicating Cushing's disease. Am J Med Sci 273:273–277

Essman WB (ed) (1978) Serotonin in health and disease. In: The central nervous system vol III. Spectrum Publ., New York

Fachnie JD, Zafar MS, Mellinger RC, Chason JL, Kahkonen DM (1980) Pituitary carcinoma mimics the ectopic adrenocorticotropin syndrome. J Clin Endocrinol Metab 50:1062–1065

Fellerman H, Dalakos TG, Streeten DHP (1970) Remission of Cushing's syndrome after unilateral adrenal phlebography. Ann Intern Med 73:585–589

Flint LD, Jacobs EC (1974) Belated recognition of adrenocorticotropic hormone-producing tumors in post-adrenalectomized Cushing's syndrome. J Urol 122:688–692

Frajria R, Angeli AL (1977) Alcohol-induced pseudo-Cushing's syndrome. Lancet I:1050–1051

Garcia JH, Kalimo H, Givens JR (1976) Human adenohypophysis in Nelson's syndrome. Arch Pathol Lab Med 100:253–258

Gifford S, Gunderson JG (1970) Cushing's disease as a psychosomatic disorder. Medicine 49:397–408

Grimes EM, Fayez JA, Miller GL (1973) Cushing's syndrome in pregnancy Obstet Gynecol 42:550–559

Hajjar RA, Hickey RC, Samaan NA (1974) Adrenal cortical carcinoma. Cancer 35:549–554

Hamwi GJ, Gwinup G, Mostow JH, Besch PK (1963) Activation of testicular adrenal rest tissue by prolonged excessive ACTH production. J Clin Endocrinol Metab 23:861–869

Heinbecker P (1944) Pathogenesis of Cushing's syndrome. Medicine 23:225–247

Herbst AL (1974) Exogenous hormones in pregnancy. Clin Obstet Gynecol 14:37–50

Himsworth RL, Bloomfield GA, Coombes RC, Ellison M, Gilkes JJH, Lowry PJ, Setchell KDR, Slavin G, Rees LH (1977) "Big ACTH" and calcitonin in an ectopic hormone-secreting tumor of liver. Clin Endocrinol 7:45–62

Himsworth RL, Lewis JG, Rees LH (1978) A possible ACTH-secreting tumour of the pituitary developing in a conventionally treated case of Addison's disease. Clin Endocrinol 9:131–139

Hirata Y, Sakamoto N, Yamamoto N, Hirata Y, Nakai Y, Endo J, Tanaka A, Nakamura M (1975) Studies on ectopic ACTH-producing tumors. Cancer 35:1430–1437

Holub DA, Katz FH (1961) A possible etiologic link between Cushing's syndrome and visceral malignancy. Clin Res 9:194 (Abstract)

Hopwood NJ, Kenny FM (1977) Incidence of Nelson's syndrome after adrenalectomy for Cushing's disease in children. Am J Dis Child 131:1353–1356

Horai T, Nishihara H, Tateishi R, Matsuda M, Hattori S (1973) Oat-cell carcinoma of the lung simultaneously producing ACTH and serotonin. J Clin Endocrinol Metab 37:212–219

Horvath E, Kovacs K (1978) Silent pituitary adenomas. Lab Invest 38:348–349

Horvath E, Kovacs K, Killinger DW, Smyth HS, Platts ME, Singer W (1980) Silent corticotropic adenomas of the human pituitary gland: A histologic, immunocytologic, and ultrastructural study. Am J Pathol 98:617–638

Hund WA, Majchrowicz E (1974) Alterations in the turnover of brain norepinephrine and dopamine in alcohol-dependent rats. J Neurochem 23:549–552

Hutter AM, Kayhoe DE (1966) Adrenal cortical carcinoma. Am J Med 41:572–580

Jara-Albarran A, Bayort J, Caballero Portillo Laborda J, Sampedro M, Cure C, Palacios Mateos JM (1979) Probable pituitary adenoma with adrenocorticotropin hypersecretion (corticotropinoma) secondary to Addison's disease. J Clin Endocrinol Metab 49:236–241

Jeffcoate WJ, Silverstone JT, Edwards CRW, Besser GM (1979) Psychiatric manifestations of Cushing's syndrome: Response to lowering of plasma cortisol. Quar J Med 191:465–472

Jenkins JS, Connolly J (1968) Adrenocortical response to ethanol in man. Br Med J II:804–805

Kammer H, Barter M (1979) Spontaneous remission of Cushing's disease. Am J Med 67:519–523

Karoum F, Majchrowicz E, Wyatt RJ (1976) Brain concentrations of biogenic amine metabolites in acutely treated and ethanol-dependent rats. J Pharmacol 56:403–411

Kovacs K, Horvath E, Bayley TA, Hassaram ST, Ezrin C (1978) Silent corticotrophic cell adenoma with lysosomal accumulation and crinophagy. Am J Med 64:492–499

Kovacs K, Ilse G, Ryan N, Horvath E, Chen HJ, Walfish PG (1979) Pituitary prolactin cell hyperplasia. Lab Invest 40:266, Annual Meeting (Abstract)

Kovacs K, Rayn N, Horvath E, Ezrin C, Penz G (1978) Prolactin cell adenomas of the human pituitary. Morphologic features of prolactin cells in the nontumorous portions of the anterior lobe. Horm Metab Res 10:409–412

Krakoff L, Nicolis G, Amsel B (1975) Pathogenesis of hypertension in Cushing's syndrome. Am J Med 58:216–220

Kreines K, DeVaux WD (1971) Neonatal adrenal insufficiency associated with maternal Cushing's syndrome. Pediatrics 47:516–519

Krieger DT (1978) Endocrine processes and serotonin. In: Essman WB (ed) Serotonin in health and disease. The central nervous system, vol III. Spectrum Publ., New York, pp 51–67

Krieger DT (1978) The central nervous system and Cushing's disease. Med Clin North Am 62:261–268

Krieger DT, Glick SM (1974) Sleep EEG stages and plasma growth hormone concentration in states of endogenous and exogenous hypercortisolemia or ACTH elevation. J Clin Endocrinol Metab 39:986–1000

Krieger DT, Samojlik E, Bardin CW (1978) Cortisol and androgen secretion in a case of Nelson's syndrome and paratesticular tumors: Response to cyproheptadine therapy. J Clin Endocrinol Metab 47:837–844

Lahti RA (1975) Alcohol aldehydes and biogenic amines. In: Majchrowicz E (ed) Biochemical pharmacology of ethanol. Plenum Press, New York, pp 239–253

Lamberts SWJ, Klijn JGM, deJong FH, Birgenhager JC (1979) Hormone secretion in alcohol-induced pseudo-Cushing's syndrome. JAMA 242:1640–1643

Law DH, Liddle GW, Scott HW Jr, Tauber SD (1965) Ectopic production of multiple hormones (ACTH, MSH and gastrin) by a single malignant tumor. N Engl J Med 273:292–296

Levine R, Smith M (1960) Cushing's syndrome. In: Astwood EB (ed) Clinical endocrinology, vol I. Grune and Stratton, New York, pp 344–353

Liberman B, Wajchenberg BL, Tambascia MA, Mesquita CH (1976) Periodic remission in Cushing's disease with paradoxical dexamethasone response: An expression of periodic hormonogenesis. J Clin Endocrinol Metab 43:913–918

Liddle GW, Nicholson WE, Island DP, Orth DN, Abe K, Lowder SC (1969) Clinical and laboratory studies of ectopic hormonal syndromes. Recent Prog Horm Res 25:283–314

Liggins GC, Howie RN (1972) A controlled trial of antepartum glucocorticoid treatment for prevention of the respiratory distress syndrome in premature infants. Pediatrics 50:515–525

Lipsett MB, Hertz R, Ross GT (1963) Clinical and pathophysiologic aspects of adrenocortical carcinoma. Am J Med 35:374–361

Lipsett MB, Wilson H (1962) Adrenal cortical cancer: Steroid biosynthesis and metabolism evaluated by urinary metabolites. J Clin Endocrinol Metab 22:906–915

Ludecke D, Kautzky R, Seager W, Schrader D (1976) Selective removal of hypersecreting pituitary adenomas. Acta Neurochir (Wien) 35:27–42

MacErlean DP, Doyle FH (1976) The pituitary fossa in Cushing's syndrome. A retrospective analysis of 93 patients. Br J Radiol 49:820

Maschler I, Rosenmann E, Ehrenfeld EN (1979) Ectopic functioning adrenocorticomyelolipoma in longstanding Nelson's syndrome. Clin Endocrinol 10:493–498

Mason AMS, Ratcliffe JG, Buckle RM, Mason AS (1972) ACTH secretion by bronchial carcinoid tumours. Clin Endocrinol 1:3–25

McArthur RG, Cloutier MD, Hayles AD, Sprague RG (1972) Cushing's disease in children. Mayo Clin Proc 47:318–326

McKeel DW, Jacobs LS (1977) Non-adenomatous pituitary mammotroph hyperplasia in patients with pathologic hyperprolactinemia. Endocrine Soc. 59th Ann. Meeting, vol 136 p 124 (Abstract)

Meador CK, Liddle GW, Island DP, Nicholson WE, Lucas CP, Nukton JG, Luetscher JA (1962) Cause of Cushing's syndrome in patients with tumors arising from "nonendocrine" tissue. J Clin Endocrinol Metab 22:693–703

Melby J (1972) Identifying the adrenal lesion in primary aldosteronism. Ann Intern Med 76:1039–1041

Moore JN, Steiss J, Nicholson WE, Orth DN (1979) A case of pituitary adrenocorticotropin-dependent Cushing's syndrome in the horse. Endocrinology 104:576–582

Moore TJ, Dluhy RG, Williams GH, Cain JP (1976) Nelson's syndrome: Frequency, prognosis and effect of prior pituitary irradiation. Ann Intern Med 85:731–734

Morse WJ, Kerenyi N, Nelson DH (1967) Prolonged hyperadrenocorticotrophism and pigmentation associated with bronchial carcinoid tumour. Can Med Assoc J 96:104–109

Mosonyi L, Szilagyi G, Graf L, Palasthy E, Szatloczky E (1971) Bronchial oat cell cancer producing ACTH, serotonin and catecholamine. Acta Med Acad Sci Hung 28:145–154

Nabarro JDN (1977) ACTH-secreting pituitary tumours. J R Coll Physicians Lond 11:363–375

Nelson DH, Meakin JW, Dealy JB Jr, Matson DD, Emerson K Jr, Thorn GW (1958) ACTH-producing tumor of the pituitary gland. N Engl J Med 259:161–164

Neville AM, Symington T (1967) The pathology of the adrenal gland in Cushing's syndrome. J Pathol 93:19–35

Nichols J, Warren JC, Mantz FA (1962) ACTH-like excretion from carcinoma of the ovary. JAMA. 182:713–718

O'Neal LW, Kipnis DM, Luse SA, Lacy PE, Jarett L (1968) Secretion of various endocrine substances by ACTH-secreting tumors—gastrin, melanotropin, norepinephrine, serotonin, parathormone, vasopressin, glucagon. Cancer 21:1218–1232

Ovlisen B, Anderson HJ (1966) Spontaneous remission in a case of Cushing's syndrome presumably due to adrenal tumor. J Clin Endocrinol Metab 26:294–298

Parra A, Cruz-Krohn J (1966) Intercurrent Cushing's syndrome and pregnancy. Am J Med 40:961–966

Pauli BLU, Rossi GL, Straub R (1974) Zwischenzelladenom der Hypophysis mit Cushing-ähnlicher Symptomatologie beim Pferd. Vet Pathol 11:417–429

Pearse AGE (1977) The diffuse neuroendocrine system and the APUD concept: Related endocrine peptides in brain, intestine, pituitary, placenta, and anuran cutaneous glands. Med Biol 55:115–125

Plotz CM, Knowlton AI, Ragan C (1952) The natural history of Cushing's syndrome. Am J Med 13:597–616

Pratt HJ, Sawin CT, Melby JC (1974) Remission of Cushing's disease after administration of adrenocorticotropin. Am J Med 57:949–952

Queiroz LD, Facure NO, Facure JJ, Modesto NP, Faria JL (1975) Pituitary carcinoma with liver metastases with Cushing's syndrome. Arch Pathol 99:32–35

Rees LH, Besser GM, Jeffcoate WJ, Goldie DJ, Marks VJ (1977) Alcohol-induced pseudo-Cushing's syndrome. Lancet I:726–728

Rees LH, Bloomfield GA, Rees GM, Corrin B, Franks LM, Ratcliffe JG (1974) Multiple hormones in a bronchial tumour. J Clin Endocrinol Metab 38:1090–1097

Roosevelt TS, Ruhmann-Wennhold A, Nelson DH (1973) Adrenal corticosteroid effects upon rat brain mitochondrial metabolism. Endocrinology 93:619–625

Rosenberg EM, Hahn TJ, Orth DN, Deftos LJ, Tanaka K (1978) ACTH-secreting medullary carcinoma of the thyroid presenting as severe idiopathic osteoporosis and senile purpura: report of a case and review of the literature. J Clin Endocrinol Metab 47:255–262

Rovit RL, Berry R (1965) Cushing's syndrome and the hypophysis. A reevaluation of pituitary tumors and hyperadrenalism. J Neurosurg 23:270–295

Rovit RL, Duane TD (1969) Cushing's syndrome and pituitary tumors. Am J Med 46:416–427

Ruder HJ, Loriaux DL, Lipsett MB (1974) Severe osteopenia in young adults associated with Cushing's syndrome due to micronodular adrenal disease. J Clin Endocrinol Metab 39:1138–1147

Saeger W (1974) Zur Ultrastruktur der hyperplastischen und adenomatösen ACTH-Zellen beim Cushing-Syndrom hypothalamisch-hypophysärer Genese. Virchows Arch [Pathol Anat] 362:73–88

Saeger W (1977) Die Morphologie der paraadenomatösen Adenohypophyse. Virchows Arch [Pathol Anat] 372:299–314

Salassa R, Laws ER, Carpenter PC, Northcutt RC (1978) Transsphenoidal removal of pituitary microadenoma in Cushing's disease. Mayo Clin Proc 53:24–28

Schatz M, Patterson R, Zeitz S, O'Rourke J, Melam H (1975) Corticosteroid therapy for the pregnant asthmatic patient. JAMA 233:804–807

Schechter RD, Stabenfeldt GH, Gribble DJ, Ling GV (1973) Treatment of Cushing's syndrome in the dog with an adrenocorticolytic agent (o, p DDD). JAMA 162:629–639

Schteingart DE, Tsao HS (1980) Coexistence of pituitary adrenocorticotropin-dependent Cushing's syndrome with a solitary adrenal adenoma. J Clin Endocrinol Metab 50:961–966

Sheldon WH, Golde A, Bonde GK (1954) Cushing's syndrome produced by a pituitary basophil carcinoma with hepatic metastases. Am J Med 17:134–142

Smals AG, Kloppenburg PW, N jo KT, Knoben M, Ruland CM (1976) Alcohol-induced cushingoid syndrome. Br Med J IV:1298

Soffer LJ, Iannaccone A, Gabrilove JL (1961) Cushing's syndrome. Am J Med 30:129–146

Spark RF, Connolly PB, Gluckin DS, White R, Sacks B, Landsberg L (1979) ACTH secretion from a functioning pheochromocytoma. N Engl J Med 301:416–418

Starr AM (1952) Personality changes in Cushing's syndrome. J Clin Endocrinol Metab 12:502–505

Strickland AL, Underwood LE, Voina SJ, French FS, VanWyk JJ (1972) Growth retardation in Cushing's syndrome. Am J Dis Child 123:207–213

Suda T, Demura H, Demura R, Wakabayashi I, Nomura K, Odagiri E, Shizume K (1977) Corticotropin-releasing factor-like activity in ACTH-producing tumors. J Clin Endocrinol Metab 44:440–445

Sussman W (1934) Adenomata of the pituitary with special reference to pituitary basophilism of Cushing. Br J Surg 22:539–544

Thompson KW, Eisenhardt L (1943) Further consideration of the Cushing syndrome. J Clin Endocrinol 3:445–451

Thorner MO, Ragan G, Orth B, Swygert N, Williamson BRJ, MacLeod RM, Orth DN (1979) Thymic carcinoid tumor secreting ACTH intermittently and identified by CAT scan. Endocrine Soc., 61st Ann. Meeting, p 153

Tucci JR, Albacete RA, Martin MM (1966) Effect of liver disease upon steroid circadian rhythms in man. Gastroenterology 50:637–644

Tyrrell JB, Brooks RM, Forsham PH (1976) More on cyproheptadine. N Engl J Med 295:1137–1138

Upton GV, Amatruda TT (1971) Evidence for the presence of tumor peptides with corticotropin-releasing factor-like activity in the ectopic ACTH syndrome. N Engl J Med 285:419–424

Walters W, Wilder RM, Kepler EJ (1934) The suprarenal cortical syndrome with presentation of ten cases. Ann Surg 100:670–688

Weichsel ME (1977) The therapeutic use of glucocorticoid hormones in the perinatal period: Potential neurological hazards. Ann Neurol 2:364–366

Weinstein M, Tyrrell B, Newton TH (1976) The sella turcica in Nelson's syndrome. Radiology 118:363–365

Wied de D, Gispen WH (1977) Behavioral effect of peptides. In: Gainer H (ed) Peptides in neurobiology. Plenum Press, New York, pp 397–448

Wild W, Nicolis GL, Gabrilove JL (1973) Appearance of Nelson's syndrome despite pituitary irradiation prior to bilateral adrenalectomy for Cushing's syndrome. Mt Sinai J Med 40:68–71

Wolff SM, Adler RC, Buskirk ER, Thompson RH (1964) A syndrome of periodic hypothalamic discharge. Am J Med 36:956–967

Woodbury DM, Timiras PS, Vernadakis A (1957) Influence of adrenocorticosteroids on brain function and metabolism. In: Hoagland H (ed) Hormones, brain function and behavior. Academic Press, New York, pp 27–54

Yackel DB, Kempers RD, McConahey WM (1966) Adrenocorticosteroid therapy in pregnancy. Am J Obstet Gynecol 96:985–989

Yamamoto H, Hirata Y, Matsukura S, Imura H, Nakamura M, Tanaka A (1976) Studies on ectopic ACTH-producing tumours. IV. CRF-like activity in tumour tissue. Acta Endocrinol 82:183–192

Ylikahri RH, Huttunen MO, Härkönen M, Leino T, Helenius T, Liewendahl K, Karonen SL (1978) Acute effects of alcohol on anterior pituitary secretion of the tropic hormones. J Clin Endocrinol Metab 46:715–720

Young RL, Bradley EM, Goldzieher JW, Myers PW, Lecocq FR (1967) Spectrum of nonpuerperal galactorrhea: Report of two cases evolving through the various syndromes. J Clin Endocrinol 27:461–466

*Chapter 7*

# Laboratory Diagnosis of Cushing's Disease and Syndrome

With continued clinical studies of patients suspected of having hypercorticism, it has become evident that laboratory testing is essential to distinguish those who may have suggestive signs and symptoms, but may prove to be eucorticoid, from those patients who actually have increased corticosteroid production. In the latter group, it is further necessary to distinguish patients with Cushing's disease from those with either adrenal or ectopic ACTH-producing tumors.

Early laboratory methods could demonstrate only the presence of hypercortisolism which, of course, would not distinguish among the various causes of adrenocortical hyperfunction. The first available test involved measurement of the urinary excretion of neutral 17-ketosteroids (Callow et al. 1938). It was realized, however, that this reflected, in the male, contributions from both an adrenal and a gonadal source, and that less than 10% of the cortisol produced daily is metabolized to 17-ketosteroids. The advent of a method for characterization of formaldehydogenic steroids (representing 11-oxygenated steroids) which were more specific for the adrenal (Corcoran and Page 1948), and the subsequent introduction by Porter and Silber (1950) of a method for detecting 17,21-dihydroxy-20-ketosteroids (which were essentially solely of adrenocortical origin), aided in defining cases of hypercorticism.

During this time, as normal pituitary-adrenal interrelationships were delineated, it became evident that the presence of excessive corticoid secretion implied the absence of normal feedback mechanisms. It was, therefore, reasoned that either such secretion was autonomous, in the case of adrenal tumors, or (when normal adrenals or only adrenal hyperplasia were present) that the mechanism involved in ACTH secretion was no longer suppressed by elevated corticoid levels. In 1954, Jailer et al. suggested that administration of a large dose of cortisone (similar to that which has been employed in cases of adrenogenital syndrome) could be utilized to decrease the urinary excretion of 17-ketosteroids in the absence of adrenal tumor, while no effect would be expected in the presence of an autonomously functioning cortical tumor. Responsiveness of adrenal corticosteroids to administration of ACTH was also tested, the reasoning being that an adrenal tumor would not be responsive, while one stimulated by pituitary ACTH might be hyperresponsive and further stimulated with larger doses of exogenous ACTH (Laidlaw et al. 1954; Eik-Nes et al. 1955; Christy et al. 1955).

Although these tests provided an early means of discrimination between adrenal and extra-adrenal causes, it became evident that the level of discrimination was not perfect. Part of the difficulty in obtaining reproducible results when attempting to distinguish between Cushing's disease and Cushing's syndrome, especially with regard to suppression tests, had to do with the use of 17-ketosteroids as an index of ACTH suppression, since these do not decrease with suppression of ACTH secretion as readily as 17-OH-corticosteroids. There was also difficulty in measuring 17-OH-corticosteroid suppression with tests that employed administration of large quantities of a glucocorticoid, since the exogenous glucocorticoid would be measured in the existing assays. Attempts were made to circumvent the latter problem by use of synthetic glucocorticoids of higher potency, so that smaller amounts could be employed. Steroids such as 9-$\alpha$-fluorocortisol were utilized by several investigators, again with conflicting results, due in part to variations in the dosage employed.

In 1959, Liddle et al. introduced a new test for pituitary ACTH reserve based on the theory that reduction in the secretion of cortisol by metyrapone, an 11-$\beta$ hydroxylase inhibitor, could induce a compensatory increase in the pituitary secretion of ACTH. They reported that evidence for such secretion was greater in patients with pituitary-dependent Cushing's disease than that seen in normal subjects. Patients with Cushing's syndrome secondary to adrenal tumor failed to exhibit evidence of increased pituitary secretion following metyrapone. This indicated increased pituitary storage and release of ACTH in patients with pituitary-dependent disease, whereas in cases of adrenal tumor corticosteroid hypersecretion decreased such storage and release.

In 1960, there were two further contributions utilizing laboratory studies to help elucidate the pathophysiology of hypercorticism. Liddle (1960) introduced the concept of differential sensitivity to suppression in adrenal tumor versus hyperplasia, employing a potent glucocorticoid [$\Delta^1$ 9-$\alpha$-16-$\alpha$-methyl fluorocortisol] (dexamethasone) in doses that would not be reflected in urinary corticosteroid measurements. He was able to demonstrate (see below) that a 2-mg dose of dexamethasone daily for 2 days would effectively suppress urinary corticosteroid secretion in normal subjects, but not in patients with hypercorticism of any etiology, whereas 8 mg daily for 2 days would suppress the elevated corticosteroid secretion seen in patients with pituitary-dependent Cushing's disease, but not in those with adrenal tumor. This has proved to be a most valuable test in differential diagnosis although, as will be noted subsequently, exceptions still occur. Also in 1960, a report that patients with Cushing's disease and syndrome displayed absent diurnal variation of plasma and urinary levels of 17-OH-corticosteroids provided further insight into the pathophysiology of the disease, although not into its differential diagnosis (Doe et al. 1960).

It became apparent that methodology for direct measurement of ACTH would be most helpful in establishing a differential diagnosis. Early bioassays required large volumes of plasma to obtain requisite sensitivity. However, in 1960, Lipscomb and Nelson introduced an assay that required 10 ml plasma, although it was still difficult to perform repeated determinations in clinical studies. The advent of the ACTH radioimmunoassay (Yalow et al. 1964; Berson and Yalow 1968) at last provided an appropriate investigative tool.

The above studies led to establishment of a set of criteria for characterization of Cushing's disease (pituitary-dependent adrenal hyperplasia) (Table 7.1). Cases of hypercorticism secondary to other causes will also show increased

**Table 7.1.** Characterization of Cushing's disease: Pituitary-dependent adrenal hyperplasia

| |
|---|
| *The major endocrine abnormalities in this syndrome are* |
| Increased adrenal cortical secretory rates |
| Increased urinary corticosteroid excretion |
| An abnormal, essentially flat circadian periodicity of plasma corticosteroid and ACTH levels maintained at or above the normal peak level of circadian variation |
| Hyperresponsiveness to stimuli causing ACTH release, e.g., metyrapone, vasopressin (i.e., nonautonomous pituitary hyperfunction) |
| Elevated plasma ACTH levels (may not be seen in untreated state) |
| Lack of suppression of corticosteroid levels following doses of dexamethasone, which cause suppression in normal subjects |
| A lack of responsiveness of plasma corticosteroid levels to exogenous stress (e.g., insulin hypoglycemia, Piromen) |

adrenocortical secretory rates, increased corticosteroid excretion, and abnormal circadian periodicity of plasma corticosteroid concentrations. However, they usually will not exhibit hyperresponsiveness to stimuli causing ACTH release, will have low, suppressed plasma ACTH concentrations, and will be even more resistant to dexamethasone suppression than patients with pituitary-dependent Cushing's disease.

Despite the improved methods described above, distinction between the several etiologies of hypercorticism usually requires a combination of available tests, in view of aberrant results occasionally obtained. The following sections will more fully discuss the basis and interpretation of available tests, and will then consider their relative efficacy both in confirming the diagnosis of hypercorticism and in aiding in the differential diagnosis of the several causes of such hypercorticism.

## A. Measurement of Basal Corticosteroid Production

### I. Nature of Steroids in Blood and Urine

Before discussing the various laboratory tests available, some additional consideration must be given to the forms of corticosteroids present in plasma and in urine (Table 7.2). The biosynthetic pathways of corticoids have been

**Table 7.2.** Normal basal plasma and urinary corticosteroid concentrations

| | |
|---|---|
| Plasma cortisol[a] | |
| 8 AM | $10.0 \pm 4.0$ μg/dl |
| 8 PM | $4.5 \pm 2.5$ μg/dl |
| Urine cortisol | 20–100 μg/24 h |
| Urine 17-OHCS | 3–10 mg/24 h (♂) |
| | 2–8 mg/24 h (♀) |
| Cortisol production rate | 6–30 mg/day[b] |

[a] Competitive protein binding assay (see Krieger 1979, for review).

[b] See Crapo 1979, for review.

discussed in Chap. 4. However, when interpreting cortisol concentrations in blood, one must also consider its episodic secretion and the nature of its transport, as well as factors that can alter its rate of removal.

It should be stressed that a single plasma determination is not helpful in the diagnosis of hypercorticism. Secretion of cortisol (Krieger et al. 1971) occurs as a series of episodic bursts superimposed on the curve describing the circadian rhythmicity of plasma cortisol concentrations. Such episodic secretion, coupled with the moderately rapid clearance of plasma cortisol (approximately 80–90 min) accounts for the occurrence of rapid and wide fluctuations in plasma cortisol concentrations within relatively short periods. Such fluctuations can obscure abnormalities in circadian periodicity if sampling is performed only at two time points in the 24-h cycle, since one could obtain separate specimens either at the peak or at the beginning of a secretory episode; the former falsely conveying the impression of elevated PM cortisol concentrations in normal subjects, while the latter may give an impression of a lower plasma cortisol concentration than actually exists in patients with hypercorticism, since episodic secretion is also present in these patients although circadian rhythmicity is absent.

Cortisol is transported in blood by two proteins: corticosteroid-binding globulin (CBG) and albumin. CBG is synthesized in the liver and is present in low concentration (30 mg/dl), but has a high affinity constant ($K_a = 10^8$ liter/mol) and is responsible for binding approximately 75% of plasma cortisol. Albumin, although present in vastly greater concentrations, has a much lower affinity constant ($K_a = 10^3$ liter/mol) and accounts for 15% of binding, so that 10% of circulating cortisol is free. However, it should be noted that CBG is saturated by plasma cortisol concentrations of 22–25 μg/dl, so that when cortisol production is increased a greater proportion will be free.

Under normal conditions, the total plasma cortisol concentration is directly proportional to plasma CBG concentrations. It should be appreciated that most methods for measuring plasma cortisol concentrations measure the total amount, bound and free. From the foregoing, it will be apparent that conditions which elevate CBG (i.e., estrogen administration) may produce elevated plasma cortisol concentrations in eucorticoid patients, whereas in patients with CBG insufficiency (secondary to liver disease, in which there is inadequate synthesis of CBG; to nephrosis, in which there is loss of CBG; or to hereditary defects in CBG synthesis) this may be associated with low plasma cortisol levels in eucorticoid patients. In either case, plasma free cortisol concentrations will be normal. A discrepancy between total plasma cortisol and urinary free cortisol may give a clue to some abnormality in CBG concentrations; such concentrations are rarely measured in clinical practice. Lastly, liver disease may also affect plasma cortisol concentrations by virtue of decreased clearance, since this organ represents the major locus of its metabolism.

When considering estimates of urinary corticosteroid concentrations, except for the measurement of free cortisol, such determinations measure concentrations of urinary metabolites of cortisol, so that a knowledge of metabolic pathways is necessary. Such cortisol metabolites are produced mainly by the enzymatic breakdown of cortisol within the liver. Since cortisol and cortisone are interconvertible in the periphery, they share metabolic pathways so that tetrahydrocortisol and tetrahydrocortisone are major excretory products, accounting for approximately 50% of cortisol produced. In addition, each of these can be reduced at C-20 to form cortols and cortolones, respectively. The latter may account for approximately 30% of the cortisol produced. Of the remaining 20% of cortisol metabolites, 11-oxygenated 17-ketosteroids account for approximately 10%. Most of these metabolites are excreted in a water-soluble form as glucuronic acid conjugates, with a smaller fraction being excreted as sulfates.

Finally, it is also apparent that methods which can measure and reflect the 24-h secretory pattern of cortisol secretion will provide a better index as to the secretory state of the adrenal cortex than single plasma determinations.

## II. Plasma Corticosteroid Concentrations

The major corticosteroid in plasma is cortisol. Cortisone has approximately one-tenth the plasma concentration of cortisol, and is derived mainly from the metabolism of cortisol by peripheral tissues. Corticosterone is also present in concentrations of $^1/_{20}$ that of cortisol. 11-Deoxycortisol is normally present only in minor amounts, but its determination may become significant in the metyrapone test (see below).

Four types of assay are available for measurement of plasma corticosteroid concentrations. These are:

1) The *Porter-Silber reaction*, which measures cortisol, cortisone, and 11-desoxycortisol in plasma.
2) *Fluorometric methods*, in which the presence of an 11-hydroxyl group and the 3–4 unsaturated ketone group in ring A has a strong positive influence on the extent of fluorescence, whereas the 17-hydroxyl group has minor influence on such fluorescence. Corticosterone exhibits an equal or greater percentage of fluorescence when compared to equivalent amounts of cortisol, but this is usually of no practical significance in view of the low amounts of corticosterone normally present in plasma. Other metabolites or precursors of cortisol that exhibit significant fluorescence, such as 20-hydroxycortisol and 21-deoxycortisol, respectively, are also not present in significant amounts. Additionally, a variable amount of "nonspecific" fluorescence (approximately 1–2 μg/100 ml) may be present in the plasma as obtained from dexamethasone-suppressed subjects. Nonsteroidal drugs, such as spironolactone, quinine, quinidine, and niacin, may also fluoresce under the assay conditions employed.
3) *Competitive protein binding assays*, based on the ability of endogenous plasma cortisol to compete with radiolabeled cortisol for binding sites on corticosteroid-binding globulin obtained from various species. In the human, blood-bank plasma is used as a source of CBG and has a greater affinity, as does dog CBG, for cortisol than for corticosterone (100% vs 61%). Compound S (11-deoxycortisol) and 17-hydroxyprogesterone also have significant cross-reactivities (89% and 47%, respectively), while some of the synthetic steroids, such as prednisone and 6-methylprednisone, also exhibit significant binding.

4) *Radioimmunoassay*, employing a specific cortisol antibody. The specificities vary with the nature of the antibody chosen; some exhibit no significant cross-reactivity with any compound other than cortisol, while others show significant overlaps (Krieger 1979).

Levels obtained by competitive protein binding or by radioimmunoassay are lower than those reported by the Porter-Silber or fluorescence assay, means for the two former methods being approximately half those of the latter (i.e., 8 AM levels of $10 \pm 4$ μg/dl vs $22 \pm 5.9$ μg/dl) (Krieger 1979). Subjects studied under ambulatory conditions tend to have slightly higher plasma concentrations than similar subjects who are studied after several days of hospitalization. In healthy subjects, there are no significant age-associated differences over the 15–90-year age range. There seem to be no significant sex differences in plasma concentrations of single samples obtained by venipuncture, although higher integrated levels in male than in female subjects have been reported in samples obtained via indwelling intravenous catheters in the course of 24-h sampling (Zumoff et al. 1974). In normal subjects, plasma levels at 8 PM are $4.5 \pm 2.5$ μg/100 ml (CBG or immunoassay). In patients with Cushing's disease or syndrome episodic fluctuation of plasma cortisol concentrations occurs, although there is no evidence of a clear circadian rhythm. Numerous studies have shown that there is a large overlap in morning plasma cortisol concentrations between normal subjects and those with Cushing's syndrome (see Crapo 1979, for review). Evening plasma cortisol concentrations show little overlap, those in patients with Cushing's syndrome being markedly elevated as compared to those in normal subjects.

In view of these criteria, hypercorticism is a strong possibility in the presence of plasma cortisol concentrations (CBG or immunoassay) exceeding 23 μg/dl in the AM and 15 μg/dl in the PM. Frequently, normal 8 AM levels may be obtained (see above), whereas in many such patients the PM plasma cortisol level will be elevated. A review of available data (Crapo 1979) demonstrates that only 3.4% of patients with hypercorticism have plasma cortisol levels in the normal range at 11 PM; in 17% of such patients, 4–7 PM levels were in the normal range, while 20–33% (Eddy et al. 1973; Nichols et al. 1968) had normal 8 AM levels. Falsely elevated cortisol concentrations may be seen in normal subjects, usually associated with some element of stress involved in obtaining such samples, in addition to the other variables previously mentioned.

## III. Circadian Variation of Plasma Corticosteroid Concentrations

The nature of such periodicity in normal subjects has already been discussed in Chap. 2. One of the criteria for the diagnosis of Cushing's disease or syndrome is the absence of a normal circadian variation of plasma corticosteroid concentrations (Fig. 7.1). This criterion has served as the basis of a screening test for clinical diagnosis. Plasma samples are obtained at 8 AM and at either 4 PM or 8 PM. In view of the episodic nature of cortisol secretion, however, it is apparent that assay at only two points can give a false picture of the presence or absence of circadian periodicity, so that "abnormal"

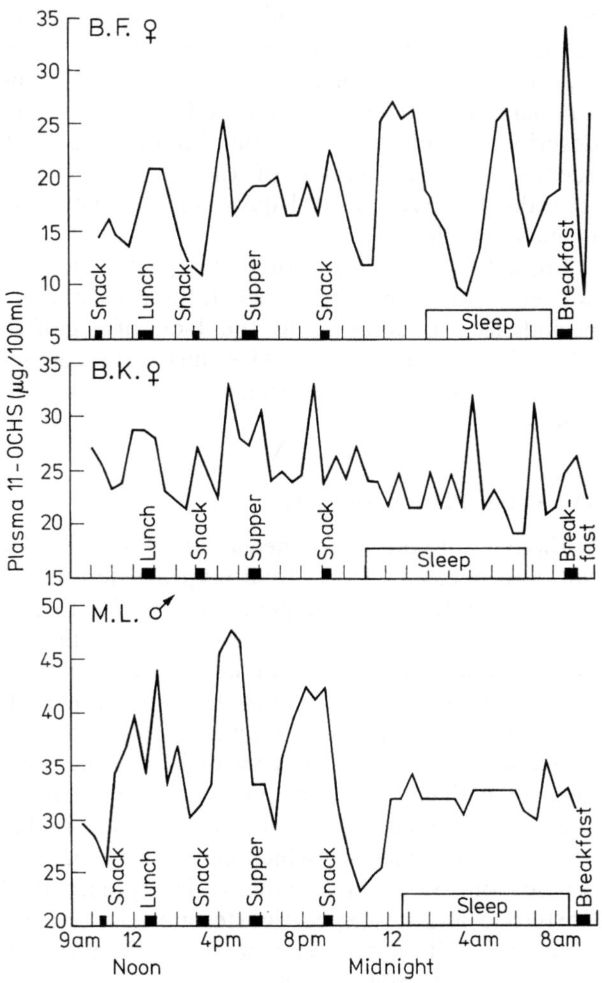


**Fig. 7.1.** Circadian periodicity of plasma corticosteroid concentrations in three patients with Cushing's disease, as determined by half-hourly sampling over a 24-period. From Krieger et al. (1971) with permission

results may be seen even in normal subjects. No studies have been performed to correlate the presence or absence of periodicity, as determined by sampling at two time points, with that obtained by more frequent (every 20–30 min) sampling (Krieger et al. 1971). Additionally, in view of the known effect of stress on plasma corticosteroid concentrations, even detailed studies of periodicity in hospitalized patients should be performed after several days of acclimatization.

There are two reports (van Cauter and Huyberechts 1973; Vagnucci 1979) in which spectral, periodogram, and autocorrelation analyses claim to be suggestive of some residual periodicity with diminished amplitude in a small number of patients with Cushing's disease. It has been suggested (Yoshida et al. 1979) that the amplitude of the episodic variation is less in cases secondary to adrenal or ectopic tumor. This is not uniformly seen in other reports (Sederberg-Olsen et al. 1973) and additional studies with greater numbers of patients are required. There is one report (Olson et al. 1978) describing a phase-shifted but "normal" periodicity in a case of adrenal adenoma, but inspection of the data shows that such periodicity is not reproducible over several days, so that the significance of this observation is questionable.

From this, it is apparent that repeated determinations of plasma cortisol concentrations can help establish the presence of hypercorticism with absent periodicity, in contrast to the lack of significance of such observations when they are made only twice during the course of a 24-h period. However, the use of such multiple sampling techniques is limited to research investigations.

## IV. Other Plasma Steroids

Although not commonly measured, plasma corticosterone and 11-deoxycortisol, and occasionally 17-hydroxyprogesterone and aldosterone, may be elevated in patients with hypercorticism (West et al. 1979) A decrease in serum dehydroepiandrosterone sulfate concentration has been noted in patients with Cushing's disease secondary to adrenal adenoma and carcinoma, but not in those with Cushing's syndrome (Ashcraft et al. 1979). Patients with Cushing's syndrome secondary to adrenal carcinoma have been reported to display increased secretion of desoxycorticosterone, in contrast to the normal levels seen in patients with Cushing's disease (Crane and Harris 1966). It appears that such elevated desoxycorticosterone levels are secondary to a defect in 11-$\beta$-hydroxylation, which can also be demonstrated on tissue incubation studies of the adrenal tumors. The presence of increased levels of corticosterone and desoxycorticosterone has also been reported in patients with ectopic ACTH secretion who may present severe degrees of hypokalemic alkalosis (Schamblen et al. 1971), although Christy and Laragh (1961) concluded that, because of the significant correlation between high plasma cortisol levels and degree of hypokalemia, the elevated glucocorticoid levels could explain the electrolyte abnormalities. The presence of such steroid abnormalities in patients with ectopic ACTH production raises the question as to whether an abnormal ACTH is produced in such instances that differentially affects adrenal corticosteroid metabolic pathways. Although these observations may explain some of the pathophysiology present in such cases of Cushing's syndrome and are of research interest, the determination of these steroids is not of great aid in diagnosis.

## V. Urine Corticosteroid Concentrations

The commonly available methods of measurement include determination of:

1) *Porter-Silber chromogens* (see above), commonly referred to as 17-hydroxycorticosteroids (17-OHCS). Other substances that may give a positive reaction include naturally occurring ketones, such as acetone, as well as

certain drugs, the most common ones being spironolactone, tranquilizers (such as Atarax and Librium), and antidepressants (such as Monase).

2) *17-Ketogenic steroids,* which is based on a method by which 17-OHCS are first converted to 17-ketosteroids. Cortols and cortolones are determined, in addition to the tetrahydro metabolites measured by the Porter-Silber method, and hence a much larger fraction of urinary metabolites is measured. Other steroids, such as pregnanetriol, and several drugs (i. e., penicillin, meprobamate, and radio-opaque dyes), as well as glucose, are also measured with this method rather than the Porter-Silber method.
3) *Urinary free cortisol* is most commonly measured with the competitive protein-binding assay. Fluorometric methods also measure cortisol, but do not measure tetrahydro metabolites, cortols, or cortolones.

In normal subjects, urinary 17-OHCS concentrations are from 3–10 mg/24 h, with the range for normal female subjects being slightly lower (2–8 mg/24 h). In view of problems with accurate collection of 24-h urine samples, it may be helpful to perform routine urinary creatinine determinations as a check on the accuracy of the collection. If urinary excretion of 17-OHCS is expressed as mg/day/g urine creatinine, a much sharper discrimination can usually be made between patients with hypercorticism and normal subjects, in part because normal creatinine secretion is proportional to the muscle mass of the subject, which may be decreased in patients with hypercorticism. When expressed in this manner, the upper limit of normal of 17-OHCS is 7 mg/day/g urine creatinine. Normal values for 17-ketogenic steroids are 5–15 mg/24 h.

In normal subjects, as mentioned above, approximately 10% of plasma cortisol is found in the free form. CBG is saturated at cortisol levels of approximately 25 µg/100 ml. In states in which excessive amounts of cortisol are produced, since the specific binding protein of plasma does not concomitantly increase, a larger fraction of plasma cortisol is, therefore, present in an unbound state and available for glomerular filtration. For this reason, a change in total plasma cortisol level is greatly amplified by determination of urinary free cortisol, making this a sensitive determinant of excessive cortisol production. For example, a twofold increase in urinary 17-OHCS excretion might be reflected in an eight- to tenfold increase in urinary free cortisol excretion (Beisel et al. 1964). Normal basal urinary free cortisol levels are 20–100 µg/24 h.

## VI. Urinary 17-Ketosteroids

These reflect less than 10% of total cortisol production, hence their measurement is not used as a screening test in cases of hypercorticism. Patients with Cushing's syndrome associated with virilizing adrenal tumors will excrete large amounts of 17-ketosteroids as the result of enzymatic defects in adrenal corticosteroid synthesis. This, however, can probably be better followed by measurement of urinary or preferably plasma dehydroepiandrosterone sulfate.

## VII. Cortisol Production Rates

The urinary cortisol production rate is determined by comparing the specific activity of administered $^{14}C$-cortisol with that present in $^{14}C$-tetrahydrocortisone, a specific urinary metabolite of cortisol. Reported normal rates are 6–30 mg/day (see Crapo 1979, for a review). This determination offers a relatively precise measurement of cortisol secretion, especially when expressed as mg/day/g urine creatinine, in which case normal values are less than 20 mg/day/g (Streeten et al. 1969). Part of the wide variability of the normal range may be secondary to the observation that determination of urine production rates utilizing different corticoid urinary metabolites (since there is not a specific urinary metabolite for cortisol) results in estimates of corticosteroid production that vary considerably for the different metabolites. In this sense, determination of blood production rates may be preferable where measurements are made of the rate of dilution by endogenously produced cortisol following intravenous injection of radioactive cortisol, as determined by serial measurements of specific acivity of cortisol in blood. This method is based on the assumption of constant secretion and of a constant metabolic clearance rate for cortisol during the experimental period; assumptions that may not be valid (deLacerda et al. 1973). Measurement of cortisol production rates is not generally available and is usually employed for research purposes, since the method is complex, expensive, and time consuming. Additionally, there are the hazards associated with administration of radioactive hormones.

# B. Plasma ACTH Concentrations

A number of radioimmunoassay procedures have been described for the determination of plasma ACTH concentrations. Because of methodological difficulties, determinations possessing the required accuracy and sensitivity are available only at relatively few medical centers and some commercial laboratories. Most available assays require some form of plasma extraction, necessitating volumes of 1–5 ml. Caution in collection of plasma is also necessary because of the tendency of ACTH to bind to glass surfaces and its susceptibility to inactivation (presumably by proteolytic enzymes) upon relatively short exposure to room temperature (see Krieger 1979, for review). A number of sensitive bioassays are also available for ACTH determinations: steroidogenic response of isolated, dispersed adrenal cells; binding of ACTH to adrenal receptors; and cytochemical "redox" bioassay. All of these procedures, however, can process only limited numbers of samples, and each has particular problems and technical requirements, such as available rat adrenal cells; difficulty in obtaining active adrenal extracts for binding, as well as the question as to whether receptor binding is equivalent to biological action; or the additional expense of equipment for the redox bioassay, as well as time consumed in its performance (a maximum of only 50 samples can be processed per week), respectively. The availability of bioassay determinations is important only in those instances in which there appears to be a dissociation between endogenous ACTH concentrations and measurable cortisol concentrations, or where physicochemical characterization of immunoreactive ACTH indicates the presence of forms other than $ACTH^{1-39}$ (the only circulating form in the human with major biological activity) (see below).

There is a marked variation in reported estimates of the half-life of plasma ACTH. A good part of this variability is based on the method employed, i. e., if calculated from disappearance of endogenously secreted or exogenously administered ACTH; the sampling frequency employed; the mode of administration of exogenous ACTH, whether as a pulse or by constant infusion; the form of ACTH used (1–24 or 1–39); and whether ACTH concentrations are determined by bioassay or immunoassay. In the latter case, biologically inactive fragments may be measured, which are not a valid indicator of the true half-life. Heeding these considerations, an ACTH half-life of 10 min can be taken as an approximation. Since ACTH secretion is episodic, superimposed on its circadian pattern, such a short half-life makes ACTH concentrations subject to even more rapid fluctuations than those described for plasma cortisol. Hence, a single ACTH determination, unless markedly below the lower limits of the normal range or above the upper limits of the normal range, is of little help in establishing a diagnosis of the presence and etiology of hypercorticism (Fig. 7.2).

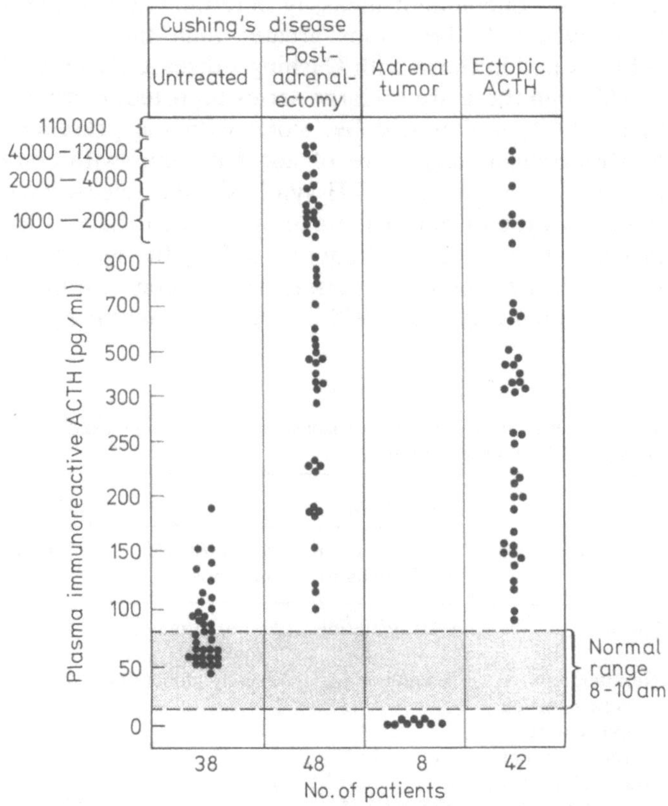


**Fig. 7.2.** Plasma immunoreactive ACTH levels in 136 cases of Cushing's syndrome. From Besser and Edwards (1972) with permission

Although the wide range depicted in Table 7.3 is partially secondary to episodic fluctuations, it is apparent that afternoon concentrations greater than 100 pg/ml are highly suggestive of Cushing's disease, whereas morning levels may be within the normal range, again indicative of the abnormal circadian periodicity present in patients with Cushing's disease. As a generalization, plasma ACTH concentrations greater than 300 pg/ml are infrequently seen in patients with Cushing's disease, whereas levels greater than 500 (and as high as 10 000) are seen in patients with Nelson's syndrome or ectopic ACTH production. However, markedly elevated plasma ACTH levels may be present in patients with Cushing's disease receiving steroid maintenance therapy following bilateral adrenalectomy (with no evidence of Nelson's syndrome), indicating the presence of increased "drive" and resistance to normal suppression. Plasma ACTH concentrations are usually within the normal range or may be somewhat low in patients with Cushing's disease associated with adrenal nodular hyperplasia. However, following bilateral adrenalectomy they rise to the same extent as seen in classic Cushing's disease (Raux et al. 1975).

In patients with ectopic ACTH secretion, and occasionally in those with Nelson's syndrome, a significant percentage of immunoreactive ACTH may be present in the form of the precursor molecule (big ACTH) (Yalow and Berson 1973), which has very little inherent biological activity. In such instances, concomitant bioassay determination will reveal immunoassayable/bioassayable ACTH ratios greater than those of 1.3–1.5 seen in normal subjects and in those with Cushing's disease (Krieger 1979).

Although there are no large series reported, morning concentrations of less than 20–30 pg/ml would be, along with the presence of other evidence of hypercorticism, suggestive of adrenal tumor with consequent feedback suppression of pituitary ACTH synthesis and release (West and Dolman 1977). A rare source of confusion can arise when there is apparent ectopic ACTH production by adrenal tumors, leading to the presence of physiologically inappropriately elevated plasma ACTH concentrations (Liddle and Melman 1974; Komanicky et al. 1978; Krieger and Bergman, personal observations).

**Table 7.3.** Plasma ACTH and cortisol concentrations in Cushing's disease or syndrome. (Krieger 1979, with permission)

| | 8 AM–9 AM | | 5 PM–6 PM | |
|---|---|---|---|---|
| Clinical condition | Plasma cortisol (CBG method) | Plasma ACTH (immunoassay) | Plasma cortisol | Plasma ACTH |
| Normal | 8–20 μg/100 ml | 20–140 pg/ml (mean 91) | 4.4–11 μg/100 ml | 10–88 pg/ml (mean 43) |
| Nontumorous-adrenocortical hyperfunction | Normal or ↑ | Usually moderately ↑ | ↑ | ↑ |
| Adrenal adenoma | Normal or ↑ | ↓ | ↑ | ↓ |
| Adrenal carcinoma | ↑ ↑ | ↓ | ↑ | ↓ |
| 1° pituitary tumor | Normal or ↑ | ↑ | ↑ | ↑ |
| Ectopic ACTH | ↑ ↑ | ↑ ↑ | ↑ ↑ | ↑ ↑ |

## C. ACTH-Related Peptides: Lipotropin, Endorphin, and MSH

Subsequent to the demonstration of the existence of a common precursor molecule for ACTH, β-lipotropin, γ-lipotropin, and endorphin, and perhaps for other, thus far uncharacterized peptides (see Chap. 2), it appeared logical that there should be evidence of concomitant secretion of these peptides similar to that of the well-characterized secretion of ACTH under basal conditions and those of pituitary stimulation and suppression. When evaluating relative plasma concentrations of these peptides, it is best to do so on a molar basis so that some insight as to the proportionality of their secretion may be obtained (with full awareness of metabolism and clearance differences). In studies performed on 19 normal subjects (Yamaguchi et al. 1980), basal plasma AM concentrations ($fmol/ml^{-1}$) were, for β-LPH, $6.1 \pm 0.8$; γ-LPH, $4.4 \pm 0.5$; and ACTH, $11.1 \pm 1.3$. β-Endorphin was virtually undetectable (less than 1.5 $fmol/ml^{-1}$) in approximately half of these samples, with levels in the remaining subjects of $2.3 \pm 0.2$.[1] It appears that molar concentrations of γ- plus β-LPH are essentially equivalent to those of ACTH. At present, data are insufficient to discriminate among a number of possible explanations that could account for such molar discrepancies.

As already mentioned in Chap. 2, β-MSH does not exist in normal human pituitary and, therefore, cannot be expected to be measured in plasma. Although minute amounts of α-MSH are reported to occur in human anterior pituitary, α-MSH activity is undetectable in adult human plasma (Abe et al. 1967).

We have reported that plasma lipotropin concentrations are affected parallel to those of plasma ACTH under conditions of pituitary-adrenal stimulation and suppression (Fig. 7.3) (Krieger et al. 1979). More detailed studies indicate that stimulation results in a rise predominantly of β-lipotropin and not of γ-lipotropin concentrations. β-Endorphin concentrations also show much smaller increments than those of β-lipotropin (Yamaguchi et al. 1980). It is apparent that a complex system of regulation exists for lipotropin-related peptides, and that further characterization of circulating and pituitary forms of these peptides, as well as determination of their metabolic clearances and alterations in secretion induced by various physiological stimuli, should further understanding of such regulation (Fig. 7.4).

In patients with Cushing's disease and Nelson's syndrome, LPH and ACTH concentrations show significant correlation (Krieger et al. 1977) (Fig. 7.5), although ACTH/LPH ratios appear to be less in patients with Nelson's syndrome than in normal subjects (Fig. 7.6). In patients with ectopic ACTH secretion, even greater proportional secretion of LPH has been reported (Gilkes et al. 1977; Wiedemann et al. 1978) (Fig. 7.6). There are no extensive studies regarding γ-LPH concentrations in such patients, although it has been reported that β-LPH/γ-LPH ratios are greater in patients with ectopic versus pituitary ACTH production (Gilkes et al. 1977). β-Endorphin concentrations are also elevated in patients with Cushing's disease, Nelson's syndrome, and ectopic ACTH secretion (Suda et al. 1978).

---

1 To convert values to $pg/ml^{-1}$, $fmol/ml^{-1}$ values are multiplied by 10 for β-LPH, 5.8 for γ-LPH, 4.5 for ACTH, and 3.4 for β-endorphin

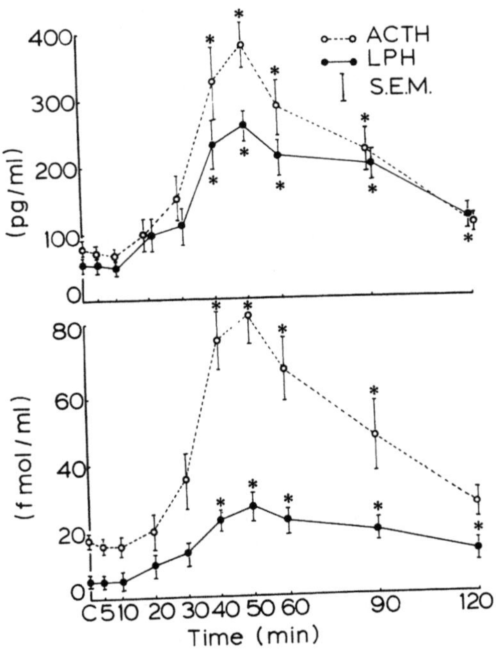


**Fig. 7.3.** Response of plasma ACTH and LPH concentrations to insulin-induced hypoglycemia in seven normal subjects. Results are depicted on a weight and molar basis. Parallelism of plasma ACTH and LPH concentrations is evident. *, $P < 0.01$ cf. baseline level. From Krieger et al. (1979) with permission

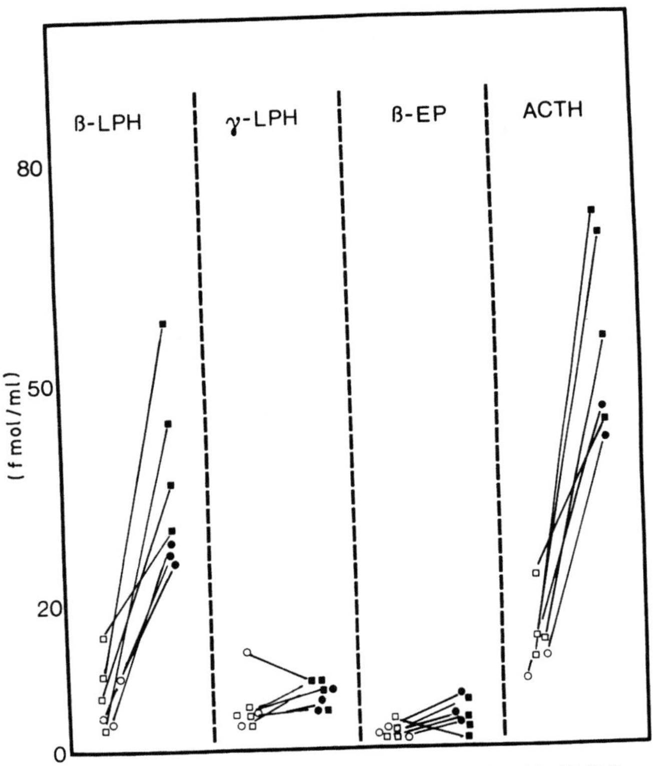


**Fig. 7.4.** Immunoreactive plasma β-, γ-LPH, β-endorphin (β-EP), and ACTH concentration under basal conditions (□, ○) and at 30–45 min following insulin-induced hypoglycemia (■) and Pitressin (●) administration in the same normal human subjects (Yamaguchi et al., 1980)

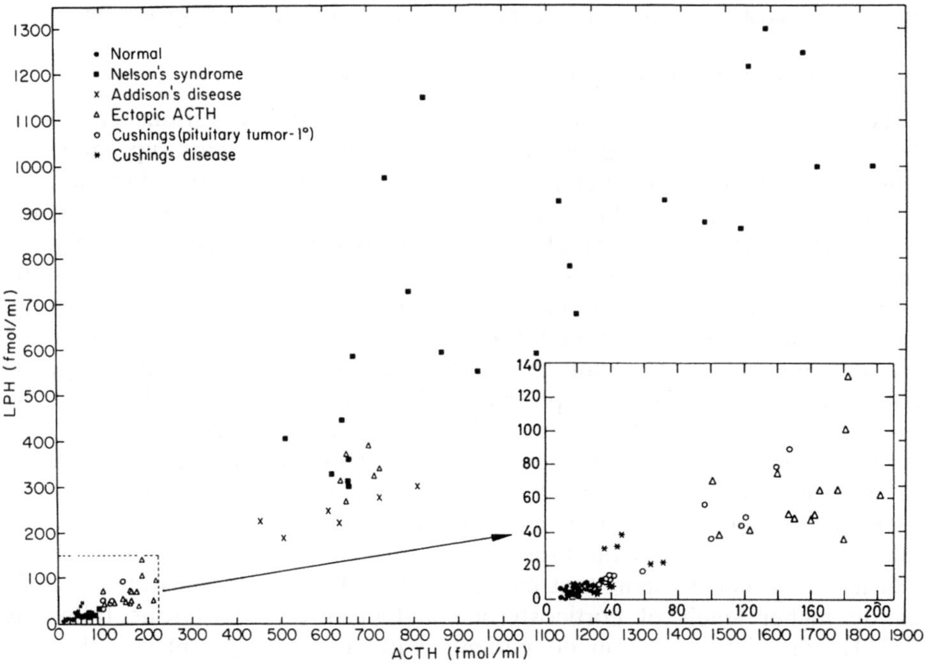


**Fig. 7.5.** Correlation of plasma ACTH and LPH concentrations in normal patients and those with diseases of ACTH secretion. The *expanded scale* is of the values cited in the *lower left-hand corner*

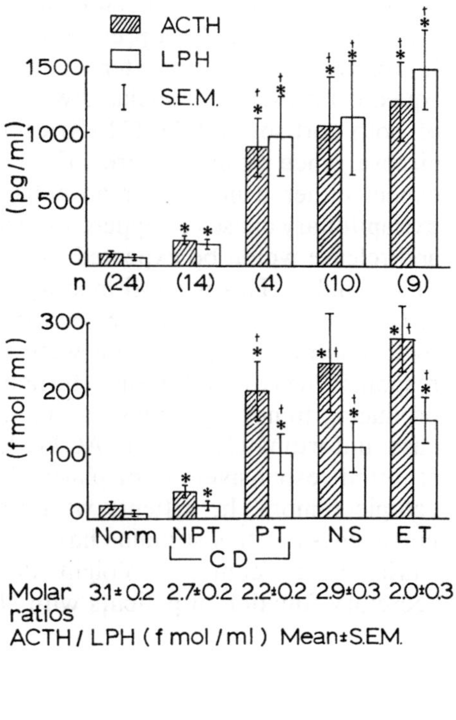


**Fig. 7.6.** Plasma ACTH and LPH concentrations in normal subjects and patients with Cushing's disease (*NPT*, no pituitary tumor evident on plain X-ray; *PT*, gross evidence of pituitary tumor), Nelson's syndrome *(NS)*, and ectopic ACTH-producing tumor *(ET)* *, $P<0.01$ cf. normal; †, $P<0.01$ cf. NPT

## D. Tests Involving Pituitary-Adrenal Stimulation and Suppression

### I. Adrenal Response to Exogenous ACTH Administration

This has been utilized in an attempt to distinguish the various causes of hypercortisolism (Christy et al. 1955). Virtually all tests employ supramaximal amounts of ACTH and, therefore, cannot detect any possible alterations in adrenal sensitivity to ACTH. The test most commonly used at present is one in which 0.25 mg synthetic ACTH 1–24 is administered intravenously. A normal response is considered to be a doubling of plasma corticosteroid concentrations within the hour following administration (samples being obtained at baseline, 30, and 60 min following ACTH). Previous tests have utilized either prolonged i. v. infusion or i. m. injection of ACTH, with measurement of the response either of urinary 17-OHCS or plasma 17-OHCS concentrations. However, the majority of patients with Cushing's disease will show hyperresponsiveness to administration of ACTH, whereas those with adenomas may have no response or a normal one. An absent response is usually present in patients with adrenal carcinoma. In view of more definitive procedures now available for making such distinctions, this type of testing is no longer routinely employed.

There is a recent report that patients with adrenal adenomas have significantly higher levels of corticosterone and desoxycorticosterone following ACTH administration than do patients with adrenal hyperplasia (West et al. 1979), perhaps secondary to a relative defect in 11-$\beta$-hydroxylation (see above).

### II. Response to Vasopressin

In Chap. 2, the corticotropin-releasing activity of vasopressin was discussed. Although CRF has just been characterized, there is no preparation available for clinical testing. Vasopressin has therefore been employed as a prototype. In normal subjects, parenteral administration of either lysine vasopressin or aqueous Pitressin is associated with a rise in plasma concentrations (Table 7.4) of both cortisol and ACTH (Krieger et al. 1979). In patients with Cushing's disease, since pituitary stores of ACTH are presumably increased, one would expect either a normal or an enhanced response, whereas in patients with extrapituitary causes of hypercorticism, suppression of pituitary ACTH storage and release would be expected to lead to an absent or diminished response to this stimulus. This is confirmed by the available evidence (Krieger and Glick 1972) (Table 7.3): It can be seen that in two patients with adrenal adenoma (with absent responses) who were studied following removal of the tumor, responsiveness to Pitressin returned. In one patient with an ectopic ACTH-producing tumor (pancreas), an enhanced cortisol response was seen; in this case, unfortunately, plasma ACTH levels are not available. Raux et al. (1975) reported responsiveness of plasma ACTH levels in one of four patients with ectopic tumors. In patients with Nelson's syndrome, enhanced ACTH responsiveness to this stimulus has been reported (Raux et al. 1975; Krieger and Luria 1977; Fehm and Voight 1979). Such results indicate that pituitary secretory function in patients with Nelson's syndrome is not autonomous.

**Table 7.4.** Response to Pitressin (10 units i.m.) in Cushing's disease or syndrome

| | N | Plasma cortisol (μg/10 ml) Mean ± SE | Range |
|---|---|---|---|
| Cushing's disease | | | |
| Active, no prior RX | 7 | 17.8 ± 2.6 | 8.3–24.9 |
| Remission, prior pituitary irradiation | 4 | 27.1 ± 9.5 | 10.7–54.2 |
| Adrenal adenoma | | | |
| Pretreatment | 3 | 0 | |
| Post-treatment | 2 | 8.0 | 6.4–9.7 5 months following steroid discontinuance |
| 1° Pituitary tumor | 2 | 8.7 | 9.5–8.0 |
| Ectopic ACTH | | | |
| Pretreatment | | > 55.0 | |
| 2 weeks postoperatively | | 6.9 | |
| 2 months postoperatively | | 8.0 | |
| 4 months postoperatively | | 16.1 | |
| Normal subjects | 9 | 15.2 ± 2.6 | 8.6–22.7 |

## III. Metyrapone Test: Response to Decrease in Cortisol Feedback

This test is based on the rationale that inhibition of cortisol synthesis (both at the step of cholesterol cleavage to form pregnenolone and that of 11-β-hydroxylation of 11-deoxycortisol, to form cortisol) leads to a rise in plasma ACTH concentrations. Since patients with Cushing's disease have normal or increased pituitary ACTH concentrations, one would expect normal or enhanced responsiveness to this stimulus when measuring concentrations either of plasma ACTH or of plasma 11-deoxycorticosterol (which accumulates as a consequence of inhibition of 11-β-hydroxylation) as an endpoint. Conversely, in cases showing adrenal overproduction of cortisol secondary to adenoma or carcinoma, in whom pituitary ACTH reserves are decreased, one would expect decreased responsiveness of plasma ACTH concentrations as well as a lack of an adrenocortical response to any secreted ACTH by either the adrenal tumor or the associated atrophic contralateral adrenal.

Two forms of testing are available. The first is the standard oral dose regimen originally proposed by Liddle et al. (1959) (750 mg every 4 h × 6). The observed increase in urinary 17-OHCS following such administration reflects the increase of 11-deoxycortisol secretion (measured as 17-OHCS) over and above the decrease in cortisol produced by this drug. Plasma deoxycortisol or urine 11-deoxycorticosteroid levels may also be measured directly. The second method utilizes a single-dose test in which 30 mg/kg oral metyrapone are administered at midnight and levels of either plasma 11-deoxycortisol or plasma ACTH are measured at 8 AM the following morning (Jubiz et al. 1970). When evaluating metyrapone responsiveness, it is helpful also to simultaneously determine plasma cortisol levels, so as to be sure that adequate suppression of 11-β-hydroxylation has been obtained. An 8 AM plasma cortisol level of less than 7.5 μg/dl is considered significant, although normal plasma

11-deoxycortisol responses may be seen with plasma cortisol levels greater than this.

A normal response to the metyrapone test, as described by Liddle, is a twofold increase in urinary 17-OHCS over baseline level, or a greater than 5 mg/24 h increment. A normal response to the single-dose metyrapone test is an increase in plasma deoxycortisol concentrations from the usual value of less than 1 μg/dl to $16.4 \pm 0.6$ μg/dl at 8 AM (Spiger et al. 1975) or a four- to eightfold increase in plasma ACTH concentrations at 8 AM (Staub et al. 1979).

As predicted, patients with Cushing's disease manifest normal or increased responsiveness to metyrapone with either type of testing. Patients with adrenal tumor usually show an absent response, although in a small percentage of patients normal responses have been seen with both types of testing. It appears, therefore, that an absent response to metyrapone suggests the diagnosis of Cushing's syndrome, but that a normal response will not definitively rule out adrenal tumor. Normal responses have also been reported in approximately 50% of the 13 patients with ectopic ACTH-producing tumors (see Crapo 1979, for review). False-negative tests may be seen in various circumstances. One such category is the patient who is receiving a drug (such as Dilantin) that will enhance metyrapone metabolism so that inadequate drug levels for inhibition of cortisol synthesis are achieved. This can be confirmed by measuring plasma metyrapone concentrations. However, in such patients a normal response can be seen if the metyrapone dose is doubled. Another false-negative response is often seen in situations in which a drug may influence the metabolic pathways of tetrahydrodeoxycortisol. This appears to occur in patients on estrogen therapy, in whom subnormal urinary responses are seen, whereas plasma deoxycortisol responses may be normal. Hypothyroidism, liver disease, malnutrition, and renal disease are other examples in which alterations in steroid metabolism and excretion will influence results based on urine 17-OHCS but not those based on plasma deoxycortisol determinations. Lastly, administration of glucocorticoids or agents such as progestins, which may also bind to glucocorticoid receptors, will suppress pituitary ACTH release, with resulting negative responses (Leach and Margulis 1965).

### IV. Insulin Tolerance Test

This test is employed to evaluate the response of the pituitary-adrenal axis to stress (i. e., hypoglycemia). It is known that the administration of exogenous glucocorticoids inhibits both the glucocorticoid and growth hormone responses to stress. Hence, it is not surprising that responses of cortisol and growth hormone to insulin-induced hypoglycemia (Figs. 7.3, 7.4) are absent in patients with either Cushing's disease or Cushing's syndrome. Although occasional exceptions to this have been reported (see Crapo 1979, for review), this test is not recommended in the differentiation of the etiologies of hypercorticism. It may be useful in the differential diagnosis of some instances of depression which may be confused with Cushing's disease, since in depressed patients, although certain laboratory tests may suggest hypercorticism, such patients usually (Besser and Edwards 1972), but do not always (Carroll 1969) display normal cortisol responses to insulin-induced hypoglycemia.

Other factors, in addition to increased glucocorticoid concentrations, may be responsible for the absence of response in patients with Cushing's disease. We have previously noted that decreased cortisol and growth hormone responsiveness to hypoglycemia in such patients persisted despite an euadrenal state following pituitary irradiation (Krieger and Glick 1972). We suggested that such absent responses represented a hallmark of the disease, indicative of some CNS dysfunction. It was believed unlikely that the absent response was secondary to therapeutic irradiation, since normal hormonal responses to hypoglycemia are present in endocrinologically normal patients with chromophobe adenomata following irradiation of the sellar area. Previously irradiated patients with Nelson's syndrome paradoxically display responsiveness of ACTH, but not of growth hormone, to hypoglycemia (Krieger and Luria 1977). At present, there is no explanation for the discrepant responses in euadrenal patients with Cushing's disease and those with Nelson's syndrome. The absence of plasma growth hormone responsiveness in both categories implies that absence of such responses in untreated patients with Cushing's disease is not solely a consequence of hypercortisolemia.

## V. Dexamethasone Suppression Test

Two types of test are available: the "standard" dexamethasone suppression test introduced by Liddle (1960) and the overnight test, first suggested by Nugent et al. (1963) and reported in more definitive form by Nugent et al. (1965) and Pavlatos et al. (1965). These tests will be considered in reverse order, since the presence of a suppressive response to the latter negates the need for the standard test.

In the short-term test, 1 mg dexamethasone is administered orally at 11 PM or midnight, and at 8 AM the following day a sample is obtained for plasma cortisol determination. There are various criteria for a normal response. The lower the plasma cortisol level utilized as a criterion of normal suppressibility, the less is the incidence of false-positive responses, for example, when considering a patient to have evidence of suppressibility when nonsuppressibility is actually present. Conversely, the higher the level of plasma cortisol permissible as an indicator of suppression, the greater the incidence of false-positive responses. This "gray area" lies somewhere between 6–8 μg/100 ml, depending on the criteria of the various authors (see Crapo 1979, for review). If one looks at reported tests in which suppression below 6 μg/100 ml was required, no patient with Cushing's disease or syndrome exhibited suppression, and all normal controls did, though 28% of obese controls failed to suppress as did 20% of hospitalized or chronically ill patients. Some of the variability of the results may be ascribed to the method employed in plasma cortisol assays, the highest incidence of false-positive tests being attributed to a single study (Holdaway et al. 1973) utilizing a competitive protein-binding method. False-positive results were also obtained with a fluorometric assay method. Anticonvulsants such as Dilantin and phenobarbitol will increase dexamethasone metabolism, thereby lowering effective plasma concentrations and resulting in false-negative suppression results. Patients receiving estrogen may also show false-negative results as the result of decreased hydrocortisone disposal rates and increased transcortin binding. The lack of suppression in some patients may be due to the level of stress present, which will increase the steroid requirements for suppressibility.

## VI. Multiple-Dose Dexamethasone Suppression Test

In cases in which the results of the overnight dexamethasone suppression test may be ambigous, enabling no differentiation of normal subjects and those with hypercorticism, greater discrimination may be obtained by use of the 2 mg low-dose dexamethasone suppression test, as reported by Liddle in 1960. In this test, 0.5 mg dexamethasone is administered orally every 6 h for 2 consecutive days. On day 2, a 24-h urine collection is obtained for determination of either 17-OHCS or free cortisol. It is suggested by Liddle, and confirmed by numerous reports, that suppression of urinary corticosteroid concentrations to less than 4 mg/24 h or of urine free cortisol to less than 20 μg/24 h constitutes a normal response. In reviewing the literature, it appears that, with this dose, patients with hypercorticism do not suppress in 80%–100% of instances. When occasionally normal pituitary-adrenal suppressibility is seen with this dose in patients with Cushing's disease, this seems to be best explained by the existence in such patients of a decreased metabolic clearance rate of dexamethasone (Meikle et al. 1975), so that higher dexamethasone concentrations than normal are seen following 2 mg. It is possible to confirm this by measuring plasma radioimmunoassayable dexamethasone concentrations, and a nomogram relating plasma cortisol and dexamethasone concentrations can be constructed. Plasma corticosteroid concentrations may alternatively be used as an endpoint, either with the test performed as outlined above or by repeating the 1 mg overnight suppression test on 2 successive days. With either mode of administration, 8 AM plasma cortisol concentrations following 2 days of dexamethasone administration are reported to be less than 5 μg/dl.

## VII. Multiple High-Dose Suppression Test

Once differentiation has been made between the eucorticoid and the hypercorticoid state, the 8 mg dexamethasone suppression test (2 mg orally every 6 h × 8 beginning at 8 AM) is performed. Again, the value measured is the level of urinary 17-OHCS or free cortisol on day 2 of administration. It is commonly accepted that a normal response is suppression of urinary 17-OHCS to less than 50% of initial value (although occasionally only to 30%–40% of initial value) and of urinary free cortisol to approximately less than 20% of initial value (Eddy et al. 1973; Burke and Beardwell 1973). Patients with Cushing's disease exhibit normal suppression with this test, whereas those with adrenal or ectopic ACTH-producing tumors usually do not (see below). It has been stated that in patients with Cushing's disease the plasma cortisol levels are undetectable with such a regimen, although no series of patients has been reported utilizing this or plasma ACTH concentrations as criteria.

In some instances there has been failure of high-dose suppression in patients with Cushing's disease. This may be attributed to several different causes.

1) In cases of Cushing's disease associated with bilateral nodular adrenocortical hyperplasia, the use of 16–32 mg dexamethasone daily for 2 days has been necessary to achieve suppression. It has been suggested that such cases may serve as transitional states between classic Cushing's disease and those of autonomously functioning adrenal adenomata (Silverman et al. 1963; Katz 1966). In some instances, however, where higher-dose dexamethasone has been necessary to achieve suppression, surgical findings subsequently have demonstrated only bilateral hyperplasia, without adenomatous transformation (Harden and Forrest 1964; Lin et al. 1967).
2) Enhanced metabolism of dexamethasone, such as that present in chronic Dilantin therapy, may lead to a lower level of plasma dexamethasone than necessary to achieve suppression. A hydrocortisone suppression test, therefore, has been suggested for use in patients who have received hepatic enzyme-inducing drugs, which would invalidate the dexamethasone test (Meikle et al. 1974). In this test, 50 mg hydrocortisone is given orally and an 8 AM plasma sample is obtained for measurement of corticosterone and compared with the level at 8 AM the day previous to cortisol administration. A response is considered to be normal if the plasma levels of corticosterone are less than 270 ng/dl in patients on anticonvulsant medication or less than 120 ng/dl in patients not on such medication. This test is useful in distinguishing between eu- and hypercorticism, but has not been adapted for distinguishing among the different causes of hypercorticism.
3) An unusual case has been reported (Carey 1980) which showed lack of suppressibility to 32 mg dexamethasone daily, but with normal suppressibility of plasma ACTH concentrations following intravenous infusion of 50 mg/h cortisol, suggesting atypical glucocorticoid receptors. However, although it is stated that dexamethasone pharmacokinetics were normal, the levels of plasma dexamethasone achieved were less than those reported to be effective by Meikle et al. (1975), and different modes of drug administration and endpoints were utilized in the two types of tests.
4) As already noted, patients with Cushing's disease may display cyclic fluctuations of plasma ACTH and consequently of plasma and urinary corticosteroid concentrations. This explanation has been invoked to explain the so-called paradoxical increase in plasma ACTH concentrations and urinary 17-OHCS in some patients with Cushing's disease following dexamethasone administration (Brown et al. 1973). It was suggested that the paradoxical responses to dexamethasone coincided with a phase of increased secretion, whereas normal dexamethasone suppression could be achieved during phases of normal secretion. This type of paradoxical response should be distinguished from the paradoxical acute rise in ACTH concentration seen following glucocorticoid administration to patients with Nelson's syndrome reported by Fehm et al. (1977). Such a regimen is followed by normal subsequent suppression. No such positive response has been reported in nonadrenalectomized patients with Cushing's disease.
5) In some instances in which Cushing's disease is associated with the presence of a demonstrable pituitary tumor on routine sellar X-rays, resistance to high-dose dexamethasone suppression (see Table 7.8) may be present, similar to findings in patients with adrenal tumor.

Although there have been case reports in which suppression has been obtained in cases of adrenal tumors (Kendall and Sloop 1968; Rayfield et al. 1971), repeated tests were not performed to see if such suppressibility was reproducible. The available data in cases of ectopic ACTH production indicate that suppression can be obtained with 8 mg in approximately 25% of such cases. Suppression is most common in instances of bronchial carcinoids, thymomas, and hepatomas.

## E. Response to Hypothalamic-Releasing Hormones

### I. Thyrotropin-Releasing Hormone (TRH)

Basal serum thyroid-stimulating hormone (TSH) levels are low or immeasurable in patients with Cushing's syndrome, and responses to thyrotropin-releasing hormone (TRH) are blunted similar to those noted with patients receiving exogenous glucocorticoids (see Duick and Wahner 1979, for review). It is still unclear whether glucocorticoids act only to suppress the secretion of pituitary TSH directly or secondarily by reducing the trophic stimulus to TRH secretion. Prolactin responses to administration of TRH are within the normal range (Krieger et al. 1976). Administration of TRH to patients with Nelson's syndrome and Cushing's disease is associated with an increase in the plasma concentration of ACTH and lipotropin, in contrast to the absence of such a response in normal subjects (Krieger and Luria 1977; Pieters et al. 1979). An increase in the plasma concentrations of $\beta$-endorphin following TRH in such patients has also been reported (Oki et al. 1980). This implies either an alteration in hormone receptors within the pituitary gland or in the central effects of TRH. These possibilities cannot be distinguished with certainty, although there is a report of in vitro release of ACTH from a subclone of AtT20 cells (ACTH-secreting pituitary cells) incubated with TRH but not from anterior pituitary cells derived from normal rats. TRH receptors were demonstrable in the AtT20 cells (Gershengorn et al. 1980).

### II. Gonadotropin-Releasing Hormone (LHRH)

Impaired luteinizing hormone (LH) and follicle-stimulating hormone (FSH) responses to LHRH administration have been observed in approximately 30% of patients with Cushing's disease (Hajimoto 1975; Luton et al. 1977), although not in three of three other patients tested (McKenna et al. 1979): In the latter report, a higher dose of LHRH (200 µg) was employed, as compared to either 100 or 150 µg in the former studies. Impairment of responsiveness to LHRH in approximately 50% of patients following prednisone treatment has also been reported (Gonzalez-Barcena et al. 1974; Ceresa et al. 1976). Basal LH and FSH levels also appear subnormal in a number of these patients. The low basal levels and absent responses to LHRH are reversed with correction of hypercortisolism, similar to what has been observed with regard to TSH responses to TRH. Thus, the absence of response can be directly attributable to the glucocorticoids.

We have not observed any release of ACTH following LHRH administration to patients with Cushing's disease or Nelson's syndrome. However, Pieters et al. (1979) observed a rise in plasma cortisol concentrations following the administration of LHRH in three of six patients with Cushing's disease.

### III. Somatostatin

Inhibition of spontaneous ACTH secretion following somatostatin administration has been reported in two patients with Nelson's syndrome and in a patient with active Cushing's disease (Tyrrell et al. 1975), whereas no decrease in metyrapone-induced ACTH secretion was seen. A decrease in $\beta$-endorphin concentrations has also been reported following somatostatin in a patient with Nelson's syndrome (Oki et al. 1980). We (unpublished observations) and Hall et al. (1973) have not been able to document similar decreases in plasma ACTH concentrations following somatostatin administration to patients with Cushing's disease or Nelson's syndrome.

### IV. Growth Hormone Responses

In 1972, we (Krieger and Glick) reported diminished growth hormone responsiveness to insulin-induced hypoglycemia and Pitressin and Piromen administration in patients with active Cushing's disease and those in remission. In addition, none displayed the normal elevation of plasma growth hormone levels seen following sleep onset. There have been a number of previous reports also indicating absent growth hormone responsiveness in cases of both Cushing's disease and adrenal tumors (James et al. 1968; Krieger and Glick 1972), as well as diminished, but usually not absent, growth hormone responsiveness in patients receiving exogenous glucocorticoids. Even when growth hormone responsiveness has been reported in subjects with Cushing's disease in remission, the increment is usually less than that cited for untreated normal subjects (James et al. 1968), although normal responses have also been reported in such patients (Demura et al. 1972; Tyrrell et al. 1977). Similarly, the absence of a sleep-associated rise of plasma growth hormone concentrations persists following correction of hypercortisolemia in patients with Cushing's disease, whereas a normal rise is seen following adrenal surgery in patients with adrenal adenoma in whom the absence of a rise was present prior to treatment (Krieger and Gewirtz 1974; Krieger and Glick 1974).

### V. Prolactin

Patients with Cushing's disease, but not those with hypercorticism secondary to adrenal adenoma or those receiving glucocorticoid therapy, show no nocturnal elevation of plasma prolactin concentrations (Krieger et al. 1976; Hagen et al. 1978). There is also a tendency for basal prolactin concentrations to be elevated in patients with Cushing's disease (Krieger unpublished observations; Hashimoto 1975).

## VI. Thyroid Hormones

In patients with Cushing's disease and syndrome, the serum thyroxine level is mildly depressed, the free $T_4$ level is normal, and serum triiodothyronine and free $T_3$ are both reduced (see Duick and Wahner 1979, for review). Such findings are also seen following the administration of glucocorticoids in pharmacological amounts to normal subjects. The reduction in serum thyroxine is secondary to a reduction in thyroid-binding globulin. Exogenous glucocorticoids will also lower serum triiodothyronine concentrations in athyroidic subjects receiving thyroxine replacement. This effect is believed to be due to the inhibitory effect of the glucocorticoid on the conversion of $T_4$ to $T_3$. Levels of serum reverse $T_3$ have been reported to be normal in patients treated with glucocorticoid.

## VII. Testosterone

Decreased plasma testosterone concentrations have been reported in male patients with Cushing's syndrome, even in those with normal gonadotrophin concentrations, so that the mechanism of such a decrease is somewhat unclear (Luton et al. 1977; McKenna et al. 1979). Decreased plasma testosterone, but normal plasma gonadotropin levels, are seen with chronic ACTH or corticosteroid administration (Rivarola et al. 1966; Beitins et al. 1973; Irvine et al. 1974). It is possible that increments in ACTH levels may directly affect plasma LH levels, since a patient with Nelson's syndrome showing decreased gonadotropin and testosterone concentrations manifested an increase in levels of these hormones when plasma ACTH concentrations were decreased during cyproheptadine therapy (Krieger et al. 1978). Plasma testosterone levels are low irrespective of whether adrenal hyperplasia or adenoma is the cause of the hypercorticism, which suggests that ACTH elevation per se is not responsible for such suppression. There is no evidence as to whether glucocorticoids can alter the metabolic clearance rate of testosterone. In women with Cushing's disease, elevated plasma testosterone levels may be present, usually in those patients in whom hirsutism as well as menstrual cycle abnormalities are present. In these instances, there is evidence for an adrenal origin of the elevated testosterone values, as seen by the lack of testosterone responsiveness to ACTH following adrenalectomy (Smals et al. 1977). In males, it is apparent that whatever stimulatory effect ACTH may have on adrenal androgens is nullified by its suppressant effect (direct or indirect) on gonadal function.

## VIII. Nonspecific Diagnostic Determinations

These were discussed and indicated in Table 4.1, and are further documented in Table 7.5.

**Table 7.5.** Nonspecific diagnostic determinations

| | |
|---|---|
| 1. Electrolyte and acid-base balance | |
| Serum sodium | usually normal, may be increased |
| Serum potassium | usually normal, may be decreased<br>Hypokalemia most prominent in Cushing's syndrome due to nonendocrine tumor |
| Serum chlorides | usually normal, may be decreased |
| Venous $CO_2$ content | usually elevated (with high blood pH) |
| 2. Blood volume | usually normal |
| 3. Carbohydrate metabolism | |
| Diabetic glucose tolerance curve usually present | |
| 4. Lipid metabolism | |
| Serum cholesterol | normal or elevated |
| Serum triglycerides | normal or elevated |
| Serum phospholipids | normal or elevated |
| 5. Calcium and phosphorous metabolism | |
| Urinary calcium | normal or increased |
| Serum calcium | normal |
| Serum phosphorus | normal |
| Serum alkaline phosphatase | normal or increased |
| 6. Blood cells | |
| Total leukocytes | usually increased up to 20000 |
| Neutrophils | usually increased |
| Lymphocytes | usually decreased to less than 15% of the total leukocyte count due to involution of lymphoid tissue |
| Eosinophils | usually decreased to less than $50/mm^3$ due to sequestration in lungs and spleen and increased destruction in the blood stream |
| Basophils<br>Plasma cells | usually decreased, as with eosinophils. Associated with fall circulating antibodies |
| Erythrocytes | usually increased, but rarely above 6 million/$mm^3$. Hematocrit often above 50% |
| Platelets | often increased |
| 7. Other nonspecific manifestations | |
| Increased gastric acid and pepsin | |
| Increased urinary excretion of uropensin | |
| Occasional decrease in plasma albumin and $\gamma$-globulin | |
| An increase in angiotensinogen production may occur | |

## F. Usefulness of Hormonal Tests in Differential Diagnosis

From the foregoing description of the number of tests available, both to differentiate hypercortisolism from eucorticism and to differentiate the various etiologies of hypercortisolism, it is apparent that no single test is applicable in all of these instances. This is, in part, due to biological variability in patients, and to different testing procedures employed and the different criteria for normalcy in different institutions. If initial screening tests appear to be at variance with the clinical impression of hypercortisolism, it is necessary to repeat them in view of the intermittency of increased adrenal cortical secretion that can be present. Conversely, in some situations in which laboratory criteria may suggest hypercortisolism without sufficient clinical validation, the tests alone should not be a determining factor in establishing a diagnosis, but should be coupled with clinical considerations.

The choice of tests should be based on their utility (that is, their discriminant function, either for distinguishing hypercortisolism versus eucorticism, or for distinguishing among the various causes of hypercortisolism) and their practicality. With regard to the latter, factors to be considered include (1) the availability of a given test procedure (i. e., in most instances facilities are not available for determination of cortisol production rates and the availability of ACTH assays is still somewhat limited), (2) the ease of testing (adequate determination of circadian periodicity requires frequent sampling or at least procurement of several samples in the evening hours, a procedure not suitable for outpatient testing; determination of plasma cortisol levels at 8 AM following midnight administration of dexamethasone is an easier screening test to perform than the 2-day 2 mg dexamethasone suppression test requiring urine collection, since the plasma cortisol response to the 2-day test has not been standardized in all laboratories), and (3) the risk or discomfort of a given test procedure, since insulin-induced hypoglycemia is accompanied by some disquieting symptoms and is contraindicated in patients with cardiac or cerebrovascular disease; administration of vasopressin is contraindicated in patients with significant hypertension, and some unpleasant side effects, such as pallor and abdominal cramps and/or defecation may be present.

It is apparent from a review of the literature that even those investigators who have had considerable experience with this disease may have somewhat different conclusions as to the most efficacious approach to such differential diagnosis (Liddle and Melman 1974; Lamberts et al. 1977; Gold 1979). It is also apparent that some future refinement of existing testing procedures may provide better discrimination, although there is no data base at present with which to examine this. For example, the present use of standardized doses of dexamethasone or metyrapone, rather than the preferable relating of dosage to body weight or surface area, may be responsible for some of the ambiguity of testing; i. e., the paradoxical suppression on low-dose dexamethasone in children with Cushing's disease, in whom the dexamethasone levels achieved by administration of a standard dose are greater than required for discrimination.

Much of the testing described can be performed on an outpatient basis. Tables 7.6 and 7.7 and the following comments represent a personal approach to these considerations. For the initial discrimination between patients with hypercortisolism and those who may have suggestive clinical manifestations, but who are actually eucorticoid, there are two readily available outpatient procedures. These are the early morning plasma cortisol concentrations following administration of 1 mg dexamethasone at midnight and, on a subsequent occasion, determination of the 24-h urinary free cortisol excretion. If the plasma cortisol level at 8 AM following midnight dexamethasone administration is equal to or less than 6 μg/dl, the diagnosis of hypercortisolism is invalid and further studies are unnecessary. This is equally true if the urinary cortisol level is equal to or less than 100 μg/24 h. The only caveat in this regard is that if hypercortisolism is strongly suspected, several repeat determinations at intervals should be performed, in view of the noted intermittency of excess cortisol production in some instances of this disease. If the plasma cortisol level at 8 AM following midnight dexamethasone administration is greater

**Table 7.6.** Value of laboratory tests in separating patients with and without hypercortisolism. Data composite from Lamberts et al. (1977), Nichols et al. (1968), and Eddy et al. (1973)

| | Abnormal (%) | |
|---|---|---|
| | Cushing's disease | Normal subjects[a] |
| Urinary 17-OHCS (mg/24 h) | 85 | 17 |
| Urinary 17-OHCS (mg/g creatinine) | 100 | 0 |
| Urinary free cortisol (μg/24 h) | 90–100 | 0–10 |
| Cortisol secretory rate (mg/24 h) | 100 | 35 |
| Cortisol secretory rate (mg/g creatinine) | 100 | 0 |
| Dexamethasone (2 mg): urinary 17-OHCS (mg/24 h) | 80–100 | 14 |
| Dexamethasone (2 mg): urinary free cortisol (μg/24 h) | 80–100 | 5 |
| Plasma cortisol (1 mg dexmethasone) | 95[b] | 20[c] |
| Plasma cortisol (Circadian pattern)[d] | 95–100 | 10–20 |

[a] Including hospitalized patients and those with obesity.
[b] If values of < 10 μg/100 ml are accepted as normal criteria; 100% if values < 6 μg/100 ml are accepted as normal (see text).
[c] If values of < 10 μg/100 ml are accepted as normal criteria; 50% if values < 6 μg/100 ml are accepted as normal (see text).
[d] Sampling every 6 h (Krieger et al. 1971).

**Table 7.7.** Value of laboratory tests in differential diagnosis of hypercortisolism

| | Abnormal (%) | |
|---|---|---|
| | Cushing's disease | Other etiologies |
| Vasopressin[a] | 5 | 75 |
| Metyrapone[b] | 8 | 60–70 |
| High-dose dexamethasone | 0[c] | 90–100 |
| Plasma ACTH concentration[d] | See text | 100 |

[a] Abnormal = no response.
[b] Abnormal = < 50% increment in urine 17-OHCS or 17-ketogenic steroids (KGS).
[c] Paradoxical responses require repeat.
[d] Abnormal = AM level < 30 pg/ml or > 200 pg/ml.

than 6 but equal to or less than 10 μg/dl, performance of the 2-day 2 mg dexamethasone test for determination of urinary cortisol prior to and on day 2 of dexamethasone administration should provide discrimination between normal subjects and those with hypercortisolism. If the patient is hospitalized or if there are facilities for determination of late afternoon and evening plasma cortisol levels, then determination of plasma cortisol concentrations at 8 AM and preferably at 8 PM may be useful in screening, since this will indicate in a very limited way whether normal circadian variation is present. In addition, the presence of cortisol concentrations greater than 15 μg/dl at 8 PM is highly suggestive of hypercortisolism. In some institutions, such determination is combined with the overnight dexamethasone administration test, providing two criteria for differentiation.

**Table 7.8.** Differential diagnosis of depression and Cushing's syndrome

| | Depression | Cushing's syndrome |
|---|---|---|
| Urinary 17-OHCS | ↑ | ↑ |
| Response to 2 mg dexamethasone | May be abnormal | Abnormal |
| Urinary free cortisol | May be ↑ | ↑ |
| Cortisol secretory rate | ↑ | ↑ |
| Circadian pattern | Normal, ↑ level | Abnormal |
| Plasma cortisol (1 mg dexamethasone) | May be abnormal | Abnormal |
| Plasma cortisol response to hypoglycemia | Usually normal | Abnormal |

The foregoing tests will usually exclude the diagnosis of simple obesity in contradistinction to hypercortisolism. As noted in Table 7.8, such tests, however, may not exclude patients with depression, tested because of some clinical stigmata that might suggest Cushing's disease. Occasionally, abnormal results are also obtained in diabetics or in patients with chronic illness (such as carcinoma), where it is inferred that associated stress may be responsible for the abnormal tests. Since depression, diabetes, or carcinoma can also occur in patients with hypercortisolism, such clinical conditions may pose diagnostic difficulties.

In differentiating between various forms of hypercortisolism (Tables 7.9 and 7.10) determination of plasma ACTH concentrations is possibly the most direct approach. Morning levels less than 30 pg/ml are not seen in patients with Cushing's disease or ectopic tumor, whereas levels above this are not seen in patients with adrenal adenoma or carcinoma (save in the very rare instances noted above, in which there may be ectopic production of ACTH by an adrenal carcinoma). Levels of plasma ACTH greater than 300 pg/ml are rarely seen in patients with Cushing's disease (although some exceptions may be seen in those cases with gross sellar enlargement at the time of initial diagnosis), whereas levels above this are common in patients with ectopic tumor production, who rarely have concentrations below this level. The high-dose (8 mg) dexamethasone suppression test also discriminates Cushing's disease from other etiologies. If no suppression is obtained, it will not distinguish between ectopic production and adrenal tumor, and here the plasma ACTH determination is of help. As noted, some cases of nodular hyperplasia may show resistance to this dose. In these instances, if such lack of suppression is coupled with the presence of low plasma ACTH concentrations, confusion with adrenal tumor may occur and lateralization (see below) may be necessary. If suppression is obtained in the presence of markedly elevated ACTH concentrations, this could suggest an ectopic source, and this would have to be further pursued (see below). The simplicity of the vasopressin test, which requires only the collection of blood samples over a 2-h period, has much to recommend it over the standard metyrapone test, which utilizes determination of urinary steroids. However, testing using midnight administration of metyrapone with subsequent morning plasma ACTH and/or compound S determinations may be as efficacious as the vasopressin test, although at present there are no comparative data. With either of these tests, the absence of normal responsiveness is suggestive of adrenal tumor or ectopic ACTH production,

**Table 7.9.** Plasma corticosteroid responses to diagnostic maneuvers designed to demonstrate nonautonomy (as in adrenal hyperplasia) or autonomy (as in adrenal, pituitary, or ectopic tumor) of adrenal function

| Condition | Plasma 11-hydroxycorticosteroids | | | | | Basal plasma ACTH |
|---|---|---|---|---|---|---|
| | Basal (8 AM) | Circadian variation | Response to dexamethasone (1 mg at midnight) | Response to aqueous Pitressin (10 units i.m.) | Response to ACTH | |
| Normal | 10–20 µg/dl | AM > PM 8 PM 2–10 µg/dl | > 6 µg/dl | Increment ≧ 8 µg/dl above baseline | Doubling of baseline value | 20–100 pg/ml (8 AM) |
| Adrenal hyperplasia | Normal or increased | Absent | > 6 µg/dl | Normal or increased | Increased | Normal or increased |
| Adrenal adenoma | Normal or increased | Absent | > 6 µg/dl | Absent[a] | No or normal response | Decreased |
| Adrenal carcinoma | Increased | Absent | > 6 µg/dl | Absent[a] | No response | Decreased (rare exceptions) |
| Pituitary tumor | Increased | Absent | > 6 µg/dl | Absent[a] | No to slight response | Moderately or markedly increased |
| Ectopic ACTH | Increased | Absent | > 6 µg/dl | Usually absent (occasional exceptions)[a] | Usually no response | Moderately or markedly increased |

[a] Response of plasma ACTH must be determined if adrenal response to ACTH is absent.

**Table 7.10.** Urinary corticosteroid responses to diagnostic maneuvers designed to demonstrate nonautonomy (as in adrenal hyperplasia) or autonomy (as in adrenal, pituitary, or ectopic tumors) of adrenal function

| Condition | Urinary 17-hydroxycorticosteroids | | | | | Urinary 17-ketosteroids |
|---|---|---|---|---|---|---|
| | Basal | Suppression with 2 mg dex | Dex 8 mg | ACTH stimulation | Metyrapone | Basal |
| Normal | 3–10 mg/24 h[a] | < 4 mg/24 h[a] | < 50–60% initial value[a] | Two- to threefold increase over baseline | Twofold increase over baseline (or > 5 mg increment/24 h) | Females, 5–15 mg/24 h; males, 8–20 mg/24 h |
| Adrenal hyperplasia | Increased | Not suppressed | < 50–60% initial value, occasional paradoxical response | Hyperresponsive | Hyperresponsive | Normal or increased |
| Nodular hyperplasia | Increased | Not suppressed | May not suppress | No or normal response | Variable | Normal or increased |
| Adrenal adenoma | Increased | Not suppressed | Not suppressed | No or normal response | No or decreased response | Decreased or normal |
| Adrenal carcinoma | Markedly increased | Not suppressed | Not suppressed (rare exceptions) | No response (rare exceptions) | No response | Markedly increased |
| Pituitary tumor | Increased markedly increased | Not suppressed | Not suppressed | No to slight response | No response | Increased |
| Ectopic ACTH | Markedly increased | Not suppressed | Usually not suppressed | Usually no response | No response | Increased |

[a] The same considerations apply, for the most part, to urinary cortisol: normal basal levels 20–100 μg/24 h; dexamethasone (dex) < 20 μg/24 h; 8 mg dex < 20% of basal level. Quantification of response in pathological situations may show greater variability than seen in urinary 17-OHCS response. Basal levels not affected by liver disease or drugs affecting hepatic metabolism are affected only by severe renal disease.

although, as noted, some ectopic tumors do respond to vasopressin. It is suggested that in such instances the tumor may be producing a CRF-like substance, and that the ACTH response seen is secondary to direct pituitary stimulation by vasopressin. This hypothesis can only be confirmed by extraction of CRF from such tumors. In rare instances, both ACTH and CRF-like material may actually be produced by a tumor (Birkenhager et al. 1976).

It is apparent that a differential diagnosis of Cushing's disease from adrenal tumor is feasible, especially when confirmation of the latter is obtained by any of the newer means of adrenal imaging (see below). It is also apparent that the differentiation between ectopic ACTH production and Cushing's disease is sometimes difficult. When there is obvious clinical evidence of associated carcinoma, there is usually no such diagnostic difficulty. The difficulty arises in those patients with relatively slow-growing tumors, such as bronchial carcinoids, thymomas, medullary thyroid carcinomas, and occasional pancreatic neoplasms, where the underlying neoplasm may not readily be visible with routine roentgenographic studies and where clinical symptoms suggestive of carcinoma may be lacking. Screening of patients with suspected Cushing's disease with determination of urinary 5-hydroxyindoleacetic acid levels is helpful in diagnosing asymptomatic bronchial carcinoid, which can then lead to the use of additional tomographic and/or bronchoscopic procedures by which such small neoplasms may be visualized.

## G. Venous Catheterization for Ectopic ACTH-Producing Tumor Localization

Whole-body venous catheterization has been suggested, since in patients with pituitary-dependent Cushing's disease, there should be a gradient between ACTH concentrations in blood obtained from the jugular (or preferable the inferior petrosal sinus) and that obtained simultaneously in the periphery, whereas in ectopic production no gradient would be obtained except for an immediate increase in ACTH concentrations near the tumor. In practice, such a rationale is affected by several factors: (1) the presence of pulsatile secretion requires obtaining of an adequate peripheral baseline with which to compare concentrations from other sources; (2) in some instances, jugular blood will be sufficiently diluted so that the necessary discrimination is better obtained by the more difficult catheterization of the inferior petrosal sinus; and (3) if an ectopic tumor is secreting CRF-like material, a jugular-peripheral gradient will still be present.

There are few data with regard to normal jugular-peripheral vein gradients. In a patient with a macroscopic pituitary tumor associated with Cushing's disease (Brown et al. 1973), a gradient of 1.4 was noted. In another case with dexamethasone nonsuppressibility, and a normal sella turcica, a similar gradient was also present. Exploration revealed only Crookes' changes, although the clinical features of Cushing's syndrome regressed postoperatively (Corrigan et al. 1977). The presence of a jugular-peripheral gradient was also reported in a case in which the CAT scan demonstrated a tumor in the tail of the pancreas in whom catheterization also showed increased levels from the left adrenal vein, suggesting a possible connection between pancreatic and adrenal blood supplies, while in two other catheterizations in pituitary-dependent Cushing's disease, a gradient was present in one, but equivocal results were found in the other. In ectopic ACTH-producing tumors, local sampling has aided in localization of tumor to the adrenal in one patient, and to the thymus in two, despite initially normal anterior mediastinal X-rays in the latter (Rees et al. 1978).

At present, there are insufficient data with regard to plasma ratios of ACTH and other peptides derived from the precursor molecule (see Chap. 2) to enable these to be utilized for differential diagnosis. In the future, such determinations may represent a promising approach in that ratios of various peptides may vary in cases where they are produced ectopically and where they are synthesized by the pituitary gland.

## H. Pituitary X-Ray Localization

This has been alluded to in Chap. 6 and is displayed in Figs. 7.7–7.10. It can be seen from Table 7.11 that conventional X-ray of the sella turcica can reveal evidence of enlargement in as many as 20% of patients with Cushing's disease, although in two series an even higher incidence was noted. It is also apparent from this table that a variable percentage of endocrinologically normal subjects may have evidence of sellar abnormality, such as double contours of the floor and anterior wall, abnormal size and/or shape, and erosion or localized thinning of the lamina dura. When assessed by lateral radiographs of the skull and lateral polytome hypocycloidal tomography, the series reported by Swanson and du Boulay (1975) showed that 17% of the subjects had thinning of the lamina dura. The differences noted in the scoring in the two series of normal subjects may have to do with whether a double contour was considered to be pathological or was due to minor anatomical or projectional variations, and whether the degree of thinning observed could be considered abnormal. The latter is essentially a subjective interpretation. MacErlean and Doyle (1976) also concluded that objective measurements of the dimensions of the pituitary fossa were even less helpful in distinguishing between normal and pathological sellae.

It should be noted that the low incidence of abnormal sellae in patients with Cushing's disease in some series may have to do with the fact that not all of the patients were investigated with lateral tomography. One series (Fitzgerald et al. 1979) noted no correlation of the degree and location of tomographic abnormalities with the size or location of the tumors found at surgery.

In patients with Nelson's syndrome, as characterized by skin pigmentation and elevated plasma ACTH concentrations, in 13 of 22 patients the sella turcica was grossly abnormal in plain radiographs of the skull, while in nine, such abnormalities were more subtle and recognized only in hypocycloidal tomographic sections (Weinstein et al. 1976).

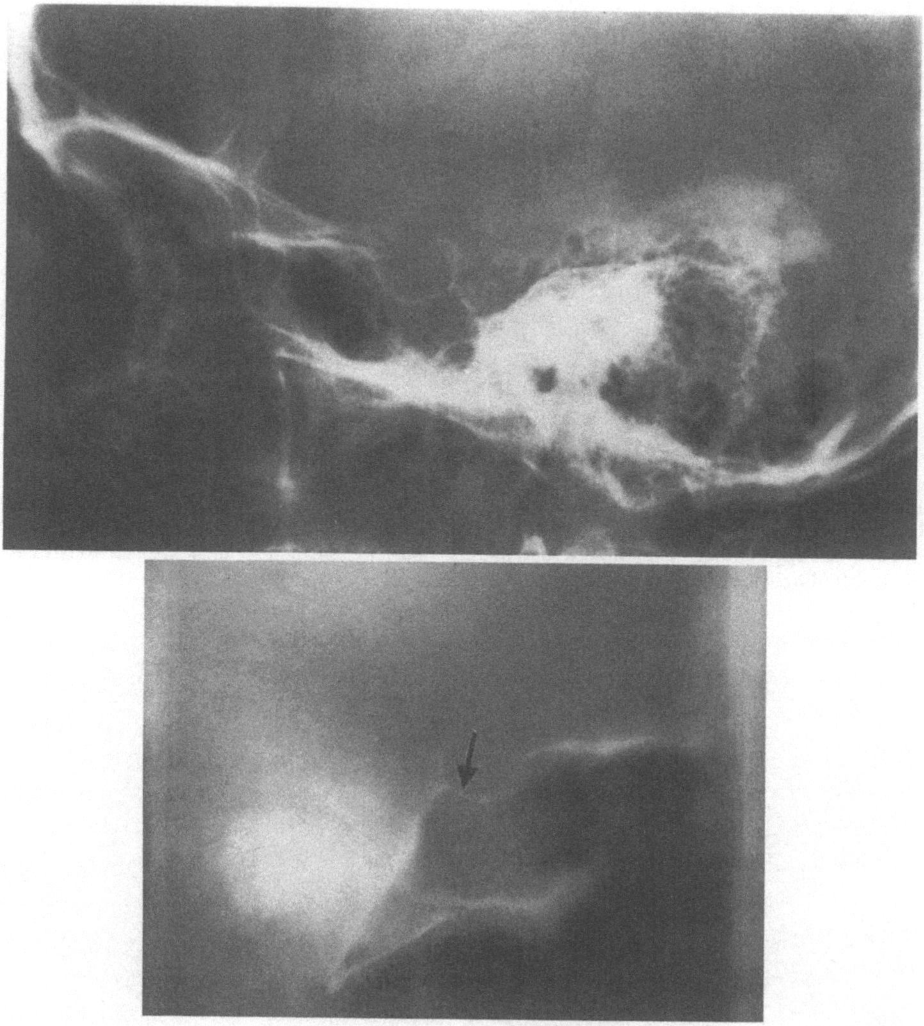

Fig. 7.7. *Top* Lateral view of sella turcica in patient with Cushing's disease. The sella turcica is normal in size and configuration. *Bottom* Lateral polytomogram of same patient showing localized area of thinning in anterior aspect

## J. Adrenal Localization

### I. X-Ray Visualization

Prior to 1970, the only means of accomplishing lateralization in adrenal tumors or demonstrating gross bilateral hyperplasia was by the use of plain abdominal films with or without tomography and with or without associated intravenous renal pyelography. Such methods were capable of demonstrating the presence of 9 of 14 adrenal carcinomas (the tumors missed varied from 55–400 g, the smallest detectable carcinoma weighed 30 g and measured 4 cm in an 11-month-old child). No adrenal adenomas were detected in nine such subjects.

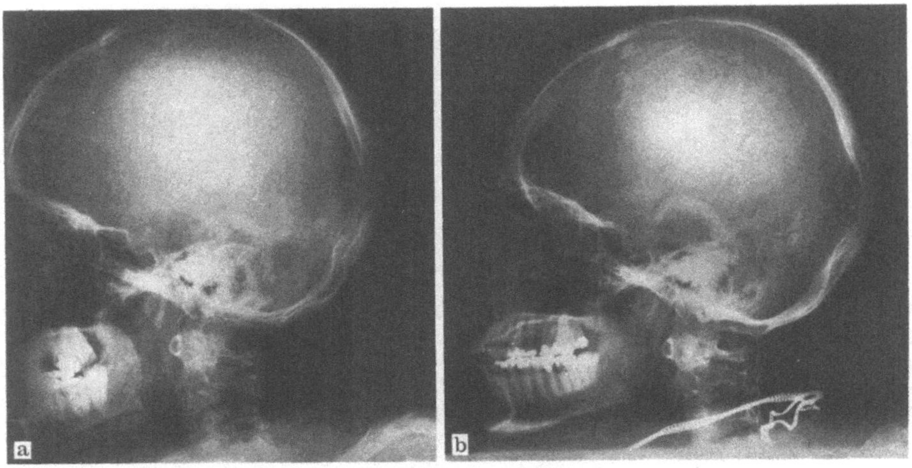


**Fig. 7.8. a** Normal lateral view of sella turcica in patient with Cushing's disease (12-28-71). **b** Appearance of sella turcica 10 months following bilateral adrenalectomy (10-23-72): Note marked enlargement of sella turcica and double floor. Patient at this time also demonstrated clinical findings of Nelson's syndrome

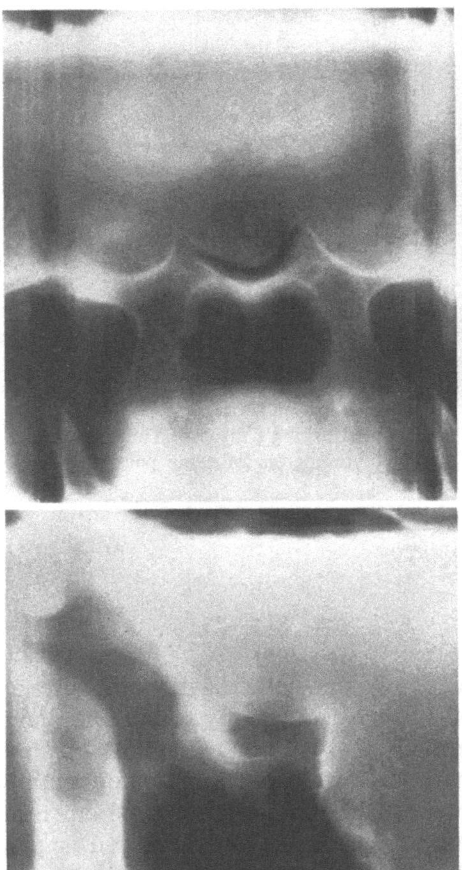

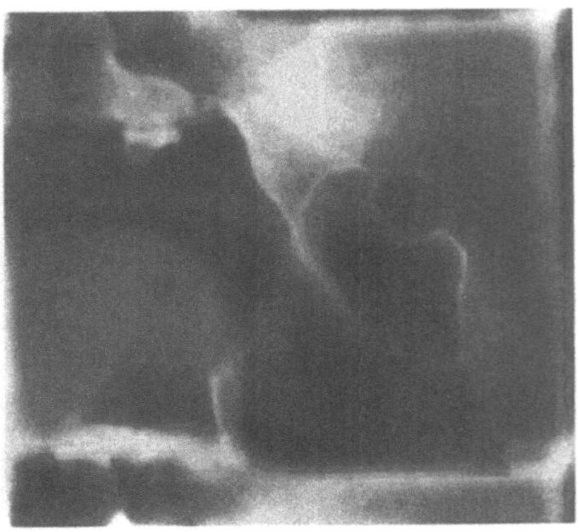

**Fig. 7.9.** Lateral view of sella in patient with Cushing's disease. Double floor is apparent on routine X-ray

**Fig. 7.10.** Frontal *(top)* and lateral *(bottom)* polytomograms in patient with Nelson's syndrome demonstrating gross enlargement of sella and depression of floor

**Table 7.11.** X-ray evidence of sellar enlargement

| Author | (N) | Enlarged (%) |
|---|---|---|
| *Cushing's disease*[a] | | |
| Salassa et al. 1959) | 122 | 10 |
| Rovit and Duane (1969) | – | 10 |
| Welbourne et al. (1971) | 41 | 15 |
| Besser (1972) – | – | 20 |
| Burke and Beardwall (1973) | 15 | 66 { 33 definite; 33 suggestive } |
| Ludecke et al. (1976) | 15 | 33 |
| Carmalt et al. (1977) | 13 | 0 |
| MacErlean et al. (1976) | 86 | 10 |
| Tyrrell et al. (1978) | 20 | 23 (lateral tomography)<br>60 (abnormal tomography, normal arteriography) |
| Salassa (1977) | 32 | 60 (arteriography or tomography) |
| *Normal subjects* | | |
| MacErlean et al. (1976) | 20 | 5 |
| Swanson and Du Boulay (1975) | 85 | 32 (minor duplication of floor or anterior wall) |

[a] Lateral roentgenogram only unless noted.

X-Ray examinations of 34 patients with clinical and laboratory evidence of Cushing's disease were entirely within normal limits (Iannaccone et al. 1961). At the time such studies were done, retroperitoneal gas insufflation was utilized to further delineate adrenal masses. With this technique, three of the five unvisualized carcinomas could be seen, and six of the nonvisualized adrenal adenomas.

## II. Radioscanning

This was introduced for human studies by Beierwaltes et al. in 1971. $^{131}$I-19-Iodocholesterol is used and scanning is usually performed 3–6 days following nuclide administration. Bilateral equal-sized adrenal glands are seen in cases of Cushing's disease. Patients with Cushing's disease also have uptakes of $^{131}$I radioactivity above the percentage range seen in subjects with normal adrenal function. This is due, in part, to more rapidly decreasing background body radioactivity in the patients with steroid excess. In cases of adrenal adenoma, uptake is seen on the side of the tumor with no uptake in the opposite gland, while in carcinoma neither gland is visualized in either gland (Lieberman et al. 1971). Scanning is also useful in localization of functioning adrenal remnants that can cause persistent hypersecretion in patients subjected to bilateral adrenalectomy (Schteingart et al. 1972).

Utilization of this technique is limited by problems of radiochemical availability. Doses of 750–3,000 μCi have been administered following pretreatment with Lugol's solution to minimize accumulation of $^{131}$I in the thyroid. More recently (Sarker et al. 1977), a new imaging agent ($^{131}$I-6$\beta$-iodomethy-19-nor-cholesterol [NP-59]) has been used. This agent (1–2 μCi) has a greater, more rapid adrenal uptake and higher target-to-background ratios than the 19-iodocholesterol compound. In 32 patients with untreated Cushing's syndrome, four patterns of adrenal visualization were noted: In 18 patients with Cushing's disease, there was bilateral adrenal visualization, as was also true for two patients with the ectopic ACTH syndrome; of eight patients with adrenal adenoma, four showed unilateral adrenal visualization and four showed bilateral visualization with marked asymmetry; and of four patients with adrenal carcinoma, two had unilateral visualization, while two showed no visualization (Freitas et al. 1978). Images using NP-59 are much sharper than those with $^{131}$I-19-iodocholesterol and, in view of the increased uptake of NP-59, it may be possible to further decrease the administered dose. Essentially similar results have been reported by Miles et al. (1979). It may well be that the major advantage of such scanning will be in the demonstration of adrenal remnants, ectopic adrenal tissue, and in cases where there is a strong suspicion of adenoma, but in whom tomograms (see below) may appear to be normal, as well as in cases of bilateral nodular hyperplasia in which laboratory data may lead to confusion between adenoma and Cushing's disease. Adenomas and carcinomas may be definitively visualized by the other methods detailed below.

### III. Ultrasonography

This technique can demonstrate normal-sized adrenal glands. In patients with obesity, such as is encountered in Cushing's disease and syndrome, the quality of the ultrasonogram may be poor due to excessive fat, in which case computerized tomography may be more useful (see below). Some cases of Cushing's disease show enlarged adrenal glands, while they have been of normal size in others. In one report (Yeh et al. 1978), an adenoma as small as 1.3 cm was demonstrated. It is believed that the complementary use of both ultrasonography and tomography should aid visualization of most adrenal tumors (Figs. 7.9–7.12).

### IV. Computerized Tomography

Utilizing slices at 10 mm intervals, both glands are seen in 90% of normal individuals. Reports to date have shown that this technique is capable of showing prominent and normal-sized or enlarged glands in Cushing's disease and good tumor localization in either adenoma or carcinoma (Eghari et al. 1980). The smallest tumors detected to date have been 0.5 cm in diameter. The technique appears to be the most reproducible of the noninvasive techniques, but requires sufficient adipose tissue for demonstration of interfaces between lesions and adjacent organs, so that thin patients (usually not seen in hypercortisolemic states) might present difficulties. In the case of large tumors, there may be difficulty in differentiating such tumors from masses occurring in neighboring structures, so that ultrasonography or angiography may be required (Seabold et al. 1978; Dunnick et al. 1979). It should be noted that, in all of the above procedures, occasional false-positives or false-negatives are encountered.

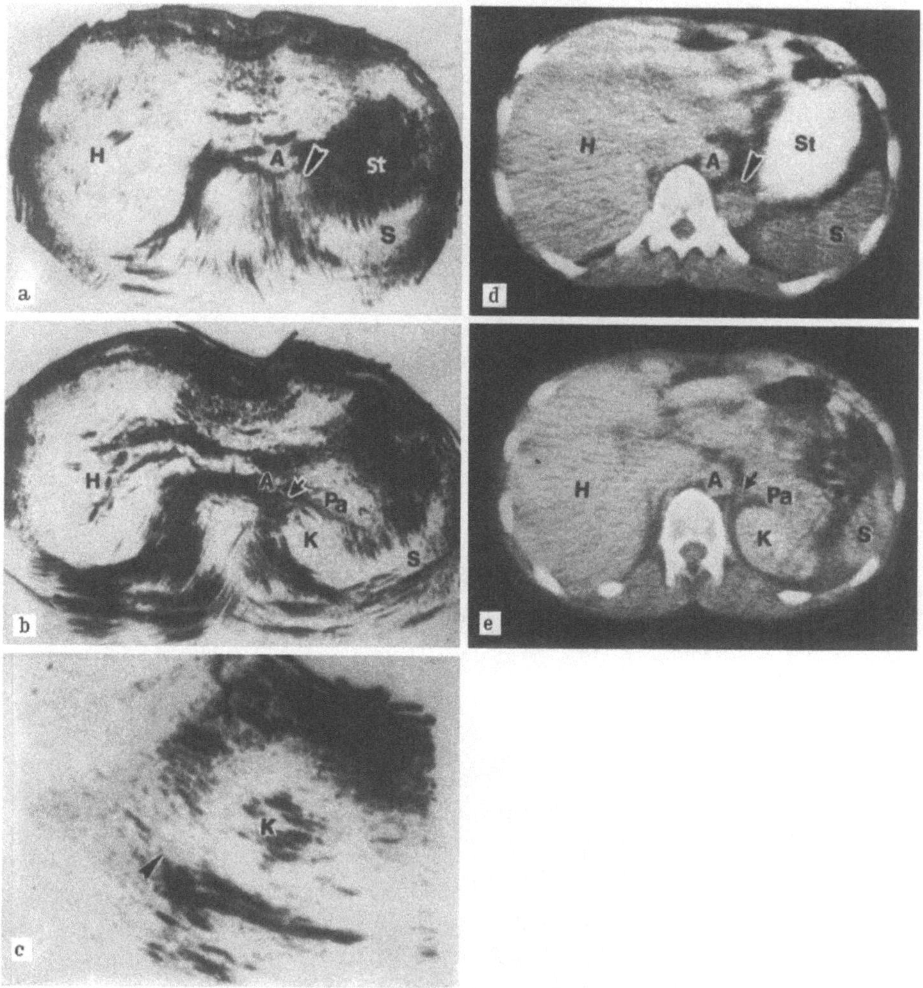


**Fig. 7.11 a–e.** A small cortical adenoma of the left adrenal gland. **a** Transverse scan (ultrasonography) 14 cm above the umbilicus. The mass *(arrowhead)* is posterolateral to the aorta *(A)*. (*St*, stomach; *S*, spleen; *H*, liver) **b** Transverse scan (ultrasonography) 12 cm above the umbilicus. The base or bottom of the adrenal gland *(arrow)* is normal. A mass-like lesion is seen in the region of the tail of the pancreas *(Pa)*. **c** Left posterolateral oblique scan shows the mass *(arrowhead)* anterosuperior to the kidney. The mass was more difficult to delineate in a posterior longitudinal scan. **d** CT scan corresponding to **a**. The stomach contains dilute water-soluble contrast material. The adrenal mass *(arrowhead)* is seen. **e** CT scan corresponding to **b**. *Arrow* indicates normal lower portion of left adrenal gland. The mass-like lesion *(Pa)* in tail of pancreas proved to be due to combination of the tail of pancreas and adjacent bowel loops on repeat sonographs 3 days later. Reproduced from Yeh et al. (1978) with permission

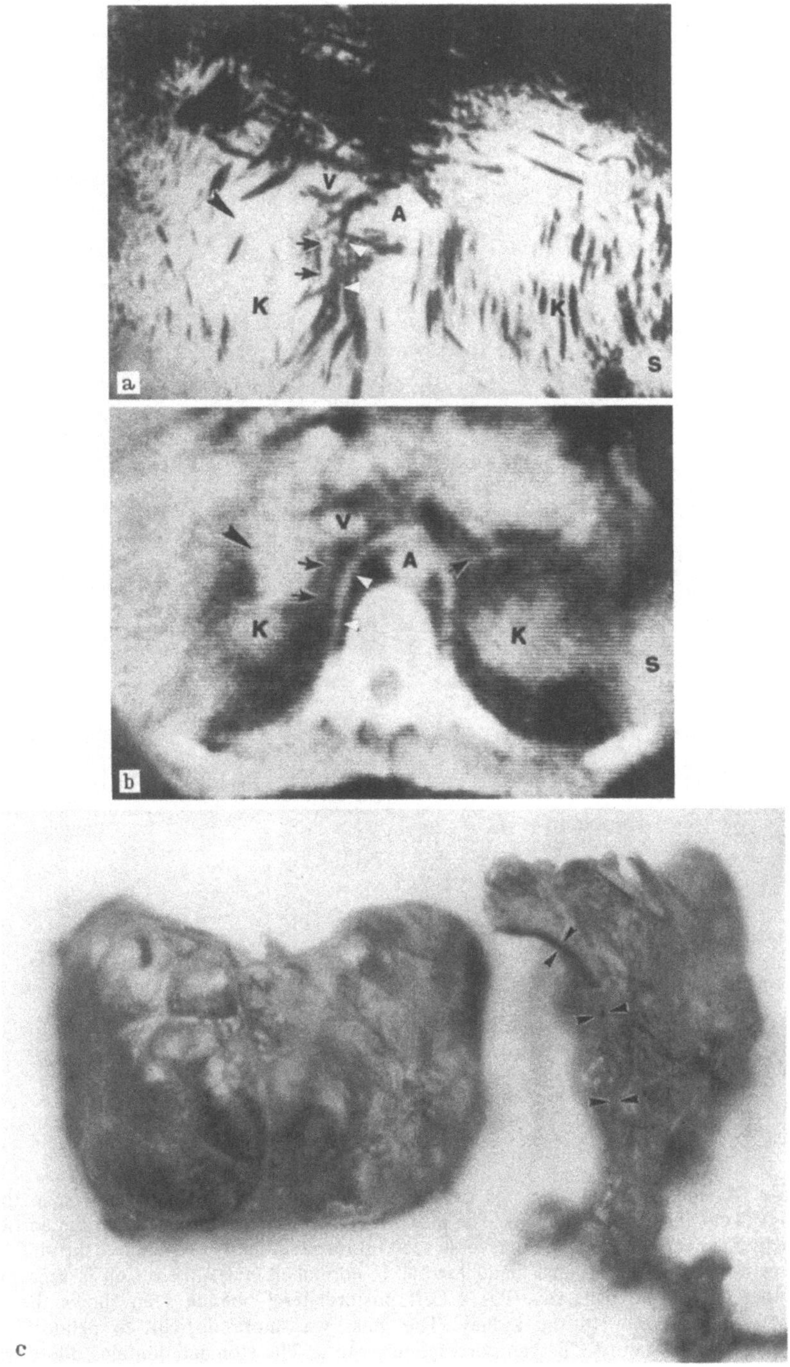


**Fig. 7.12a–c.** Right adrenal adenoma with marked Cushing's syndrome. **a** Transverse scan 16 cm above the umbilicus. Because of marked obesity, the mass *(black arrowhead)* is only vaguely seen. However, the normal medial portion of the adrenal gland *(arrows)* and the crus of the diaphragm *(with arrowheads)* are well delineated. **b** Corresponding CT scan. Because of the large amount of retroperitoneal fat, the retroperitoneal structures are seen well. *Black arrowhead* indicates mass; *double arrow*, the normal medial portion of the gland; *white arrowheads*, the crus of the diaphragm. **c** Pathological specimen. The specimen *(left)* was cut open and illustrated as viewed from the outside. Note the thin *(arrowheads)* normal portion *(right)* of the adrenal gland. Reproduced from Yeh et al. (1978) with permission

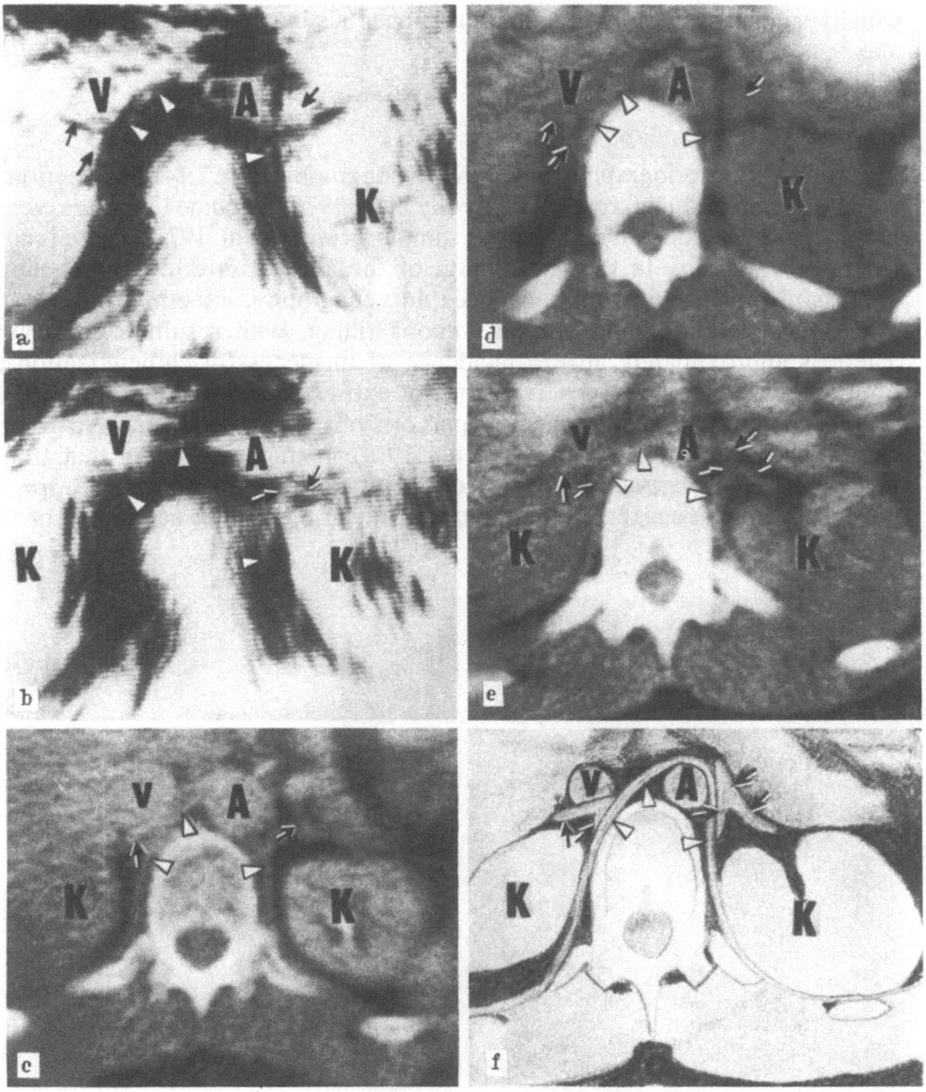


**Fig. 7.13a–f.** Bilateral cortical hyperplasia with Cushing's syndrome. **a** Transverse B-scan 15 cm above the umbilicus. The middle portion of the right adrenal gland *(double arrows)* appears V-shaped and larger than usual. The left adrenal gland *(single arrow)* also appears large. *White arrowheads* indicate crura of the diaphragm. **b** Transverse scan 14 cm above the umbilicus. The right adrenal gland is not seen well. The posterior aspect of the middle portion of the left adrenal gland *(arrows)* shows an inverted V-shape. *Arrowheads* indicate crura. **c** CT scan of a different individual with normal adrenal glands *(arrows)*. *Arrowheads* indicate crura. The smaller size of normal adrenal glands is illustrated for comparison to **d** and **e**. **d** CT scan corresponding to **a**. **e** CT scan corresponding to **b**. **f** Drawing of **e** emphasizing uniform enlargement with maintenance of the normal configuration. Reproduced from Yeh et al. (1978) with permission

Additionally, with this procedure, as with ultrasonography, definitive distinction between adenoma and carcinoma may be difficult, although adenomas are usually smaller, smoother, and more homogenous in appearance than carcinomas.

## V. Angiography

Occasionally, arteriography rather than venography (Fig. 7.14) has been performed (Kahn and Nickrosz 1967; Lecky et al. 1976). In some instances, venography has been coupled with venous sampling (Mitty et al. 1973). There is considerable variability in the distribution of the adrenal arteries, complicating successful injection in some instances. In venography, injection into hepatic veins may simulate right adrenal venous filling, with resultant confusion. There is approximately an 8% incidence of unsuccessful catheterization of both adrenal veins and a 5% incidence of extravasation (Bayliss et al. 1970), so that inadvertent remission of hypercortisolism has been reported in one case (Fellerman, Dalakos, and Streeten 1970). It might be noted that transvenous adrenal destruction by injection of contrast medium and nitrogen mustard has been suggested for the treatment of metastatic carcinoma of the

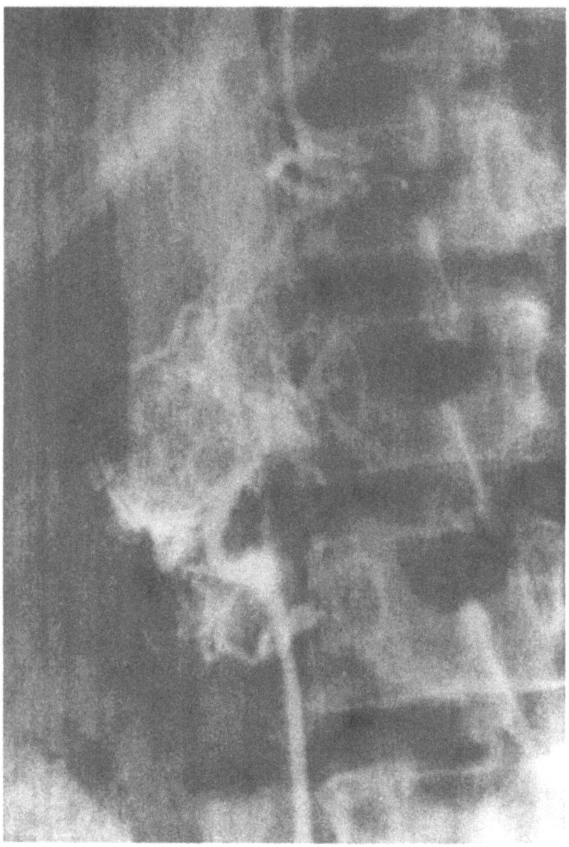

**Fig. 7.14.** Adrenal venogram showing an adrenal carcinoma

breast (Zimmerman et al. 1974). Although differentiation may be made between hyperplasia and adenoma by contrast pictures as well as by comparative concentrations of hormone in the two veins (sometimes complicated by the phenomenon of episodic secretion), these methods have been superseded by noninvasive methods so that angiographic studies are indicated only in patients in whom noninvasive studies provide nondiagnostic or equivocal findings.

## References


Abe K, Island DP, Liddle GW, Fleischer N, Nicholson WE (1967) Radioimmunologic evidence for α-MSH (melanocyte-stimulating hormone) in human pituitary and tumor tissues. J Clin Endocrinol Metab 27:46–52

Ashcraft WM, Van Herle AJ, Vener SL, Geffner D (1979) Usefulness of measurement of serum cortisol (F) and dehydroepiandrosterone sulfate (DHEA-S) in the diagnosis of patients with Cushing's syndrome. 61st Meeting Endocrin. Soc., p 233

Bayliss RIS, Edwards OM, Starer F (1970) Complications of adrenal venography. Br J Radiol 43:531–533

Beierwaltes W, Lieberman LM, Ansari AN, Nishiyama H (1971) Visualization of human adrenal glands in vivo by scintillation scanning. JAMA 216:275–277

Beisel WR, Coss JJ, Horton R, Chao PY, Forsham PH (1964) Physiology of urinary cortisol excretion. J Clin Endocrinol Metab 24:887–893

Beitins IZ, Rayard R, Kowarski A, Migeon CJ (1973) The effect of ACTH administration on plasma testosterone, dihydrotestosterone and serum LH concentrations in normal men. Steroids 21:553–563

Berson SW, Yalow RS (1968) Radioimmunoassay of ACTH in plasma. J Clin Invest 47:2725–2751

Besser GM, Edwards CRW (1972) Cushing's syndrome. In: Mason AS (ed) Clinics in endocrinology and metabolism, vol 1. Saunders, Philadelphia, pp 451–490

Birkenhager JC, Upton GV, Seldenrath HJ, Krieger DT, Tashjian AH, Jr (1976) Medullary thyroid carcinoma: Ectopic production of peptides with ACTH-like, corticotropin-releasing factor-like and prolactin production-stimulating activities. Acta Endocrinol 83:280–292

Brown RD, Van Loon GR, Orth DN, Liddle GW (1973) Cushing's disease with periodic hormonogenesis: One explanation for paradoxical response to dexamethasone. J Clin Endocrinol Metab 36:445–451

Burke CW, Beardwell CG (1973) Cushing's syndrome: An evaluation of the clinical usefulness of urinary free cortisol and other urinary steroid measurements in diagnosis. Quart J Med 165:175–204

Callow WH, Callow RK, Emmens CW (1938) Colorimetric determination of substances containing grouping $CH_2CO$ in urine extracts as indication of androgen content. Biochem J 32:1312–1331

Carey RM (1980) Suppression of ACTH by cortisol in dexamethasone-nonsuppressible Cushing's disease. N Engl J Med 302:275–279

Carmalt MHB, Dalton GA, Fletcher RF, Smith WT (1977) The treatment of Cushing's disease by trans-sphenoidal hypophysectomy. Quart J Med 181:119–134

Carroll BJ (1969) Hypothalamic-pituitary function in depressive illness: Insensitivity to hypoglycaemia. Br Med J 3:27–28

Ceresa F, Boccuzi G, Angeli A, Bisbocci D (1975) Les gluco-corticoides et la secretion des gonadotrophines: Donnes de la pathologie corticosurrenalienne et apres traitment corticoid aigu. Rev Franc Endocrinol Clin 16:283–292

Christy NP, Laragh JH (1961) Pathogenesis of hypokalemic alkalosis in Cushing's syndrome. N Engl J Med 265:1083–1088

Christy NP, Wallace EZ, Jailer JW (1955) Effect of intravenously administered ACTH on plasma 17,21-dihydroxy-20-ketosteroids in normal individuals and in patients with disorders of the adrenal cortex. J Clin Invest 34:899–906

Corcoran AC, Page IH (1948) Methods for chemical determination of corticosteroids in urine and plasma. J Lab Clin Med 33:1326–1333

Corrigan DF, Schaaf M, Whaley RA, Czerwinski CL, Earll JM (1977) Selective venous sampling to differentiate ectopic ACTH secretion from pituitary Cushing's syndrome. N Engl J Med 296:861–862
Crane MG, Harris JJ (1966) Desoxycorticosterone secretion rates in hyperadrenocorticism. J Clin Endocrinol 26:1135–1143
Crapo L (1979) Cushing's syndrome: A review of diagnostic tests. Metabolism 28:955–977
DeLacerda L, Kowarski A, Migeon CJ (1973) Diurnal variation of the metabolic clearance rate of cortisol. Effect on measurement of cortisol production rate. J Clin Endocrinol Metab 36:1043–1049
Demura R, Demura T, Nunohawa T, Baba H, Miura K (1972) Response of plasma ACTH, GH, LH and 11-hydroxycorticosteroids to various stimuli in patients with Cushing's syndrome. J Clin Endocrinol Metab 34:852–859
Doe RP, Vennes JA, Flink EB (1960) Diurnal variation of 17-hydroxycorticosteroids, sodium, potassium, magnesium and creatinine in normal subjects and in cases of treated adrenal insufficiency and Cushing's syndrome. J Clin Endocrinol 20:253–265
Duick DS, Wahner HW (1979) Thyroid axis in patients with Cushing's syndrome. Arch Intern Med 139:767–772
Dunnic NR, Schaner EG, Doppman JL, Strott CA, Gill JR, Javadpour N (1979) Computed tomography in adrenal tumors. Am J Roentgenol 132:43–46
Eddy RL, Jones AL, Gilliland PF, Ibarra JD, Thompson JQ, McMurry JR, Jr (1973) Cushing's syndrome: A prospective study of diagnostic methods. Am J Med 55:621–625
Eghrari M, McLoughlin MJ, Rosen IE, St. Louis EL, Wilson SR, Wise DJ, Yeung HPH (1980) The role of computed tomography in assessment of tumoral pathology of the adrenal glands. J Comput Asst Tomog 4:71–77
Eik-Nes K, Sandberg AA, Migeon CJ, Tyler FH, Samuels LT (1955) Changes in plasma levels of 17-hydroxycorticoids during I.V. administration of ACTH. II. Response under various clinical conditions. J Clin Endocrinol Metab 15:13–21
Fehm HL, Voight KH (1979) Pathophysiology of Cushing's disease. Pathobiol Annu 9:225–255
Fehm HL, Voight KJ, Lang RE, Beinert KE, Kummer GW, Pfeiffer EF (1977) Paradoxical ACTH response to glucocorticoids in Cushing's disease. N Engl J Med 297:904–907
Fellerman H, Dalakos TG, Streeten DHP (1970) Remission of Cushing's syndrome after unilateral adrenal phlebography. Ann Intern Med 73:585–589
Fitzgerald PA, Newton TH, Tyrrell JB, Aron DC, Wilson CB (1979) Cushing's disease: Correlation of neuroradiologic studies and surgical results. 61st Meeting Endocrin. Soc., p 133
Freitas JE, Thrall JH, Gross MD, Beirwaltes WH (1978) Adrenal imaging patterns in Cushing's syndrome. Clin Res 26:305A
Gershengorn MC, Arevalo CO, Geras E, Rebecchi MJ (1980) Thyrotropin-releasing hormone stimulation of adrenocorticotropin production by mouse pituitary tumor cells in culture. J Clin Invest 65:1294–1300
Gilkes JJH, Rees LH, Besser GM (1977) Plasma immunoreactive corticotrophin and lipotrophin in Cushing's syndrome and Addison's disease. Br Med J I:996–998
Gold EM (1979) The Cushing syndromes: Changing views of diagnosis and treatment. Ann Intern Med 90:829–844
Gonzalez-Barcena D, Kastin AJ, Schalch DS, Miller MC, Lee L, Rivas-Llamas R, Schally AV (1974) Response to LH-RH in women before and after treatment with prednisone. Int J Fertil 19:107–110
Hagen K, Kehlet H, Binder C (1978) Diurnal variation in plasma cortisol and prolactin in patients with Cushing's syndrome. Acta Endocrinol 88:737–743
Hall R, Besser GM, Schally AV, Coy DH, Evered D, Goldie KJ, Kastin AJ, McNeilly AS, Mortimer CH, Phenekos C, Turnbridge WM, Weightman D (1973) Action of growth-hormone-release inhibitory hormone in healthy men and in acromegaly. Lancet II:581–584
Harden R McG, Forrest APM (1964) Cushing's syndrome with atypical biochemical results. Acta Endocrinol 46:256–264
Hashimoto K (1975) The pituitary ACTH, GH, LH, FSH, TSH and prolactin reserves in patients with Cushing's syndrome. Endocrinol Jpn 22:67–77
Holdaway IM, Evans MC, Ibbertson HK (1973) Experience with a short test of pituitary-adrenal function. Aust NZ J Med 3:507–511
Iannaccone A, Gabrilove JL, Brahms SA, Soffer LJ (1960) The roentgen diagnosis of adrenal

tumor in Cushing's syndrome. Arch Intern Med 105:257–263

Irvine WJ, Toft AD, Wilson KS, Fraser R, Wilson A, Young J, Hunter WM, Ismail AAA, Burger PE (1974) The effect of synthetic corticotropin analogues on adrenocortical, anterior pituitary and testicular function. J Clin Endocrinol Metab 39:522–529

Jailer JW, Gould JJ, Wallace EZ (1954) Evaluation of "cortisone test" as diagnostic aid in differentiating adrenal hyperplasia from adrenal neoplasia. Am J Med 16:340–345

James VHT, London J, Wynn V, Greenwood FC (1968) A fundamental defect of adrenocortical control in Cushing's disease. J Endocrinol 40:15–28

Jubiz W, Meikle SW, West CD, Tyler FH (1970) Single-dose metyrapone test. Arch Intern Med 125:472–474

Kahn PC, Nickrosz LV (1967) Selective angiography of the adrenal glands. Am J Roentgenol 101:739–749

Katz J (1966) Failure of dexamethasone suppression in adrenal hyperplasia. Arch Intern Med 118:265–269

Kendall JW, Sloop PR Jr (1968) Dexamethasone-suppressible adrenocortical tumor. N Engl J Med 279:532–535

Komanicky P, Spark RF, Melby JC (1978) Treatment of Cushing's syndrome with trilostane (WIN 24, 549), an inhibitor of adrenal steroid biosynthesis. J Clin Endocrinol Metab 47:1042–1051

Krieger DT (1979) Plasma ACTH and corticosteroids. In: DeGroot LJ et al. (eds) Textbook of endocrinology, Grune and Stratton, New York, pp 1139–1156

Krieger DT, Allen W, Rizzo F, Krieger HP (1971) Characterization of the normal temporal pattern of plasma corticosteroid levels. J Clin Endocrinol Metab 32:266–284

Krieger DT, Gewirtz GP (1974) Recovery of hypothalamic-pituitary-adrenal function, growth hormone responsiveness and sleep EEG pattern in a patient following removal of an adrenal cortical adenoma. J Clin Endocrinol Metab 38:1075–1082

Krieger DT, Glick SM (1972) Growth hormone and cortisol responsiveness in Cushing's syndrome: Relation to a possible central nervous system etiology. Am J Med 52:25–40

Krieger DT, Glick SM (1974) Sleep EEG stages and plasma growth hormone concentration in states of endogenous and exogenous hypercortisolemia on ACTH elevation. J Clin Endocrinol Metab 39:986–1000

Krieger DT, Howanitz PJ, Frantz AG (1976) Absence of nocturnal elevation of plasma prolactin concentration in Cushing's disease. J Clin Endocrinol Metab 42:260–272

Krieger DT, Liotta AS, Li CH (1977) Human plasma immunoreactive $\beta$-lipotropin: Correlation with basal and stimulated plasma ACTH concentrations. Life Sci 21:1771–1778

Krieger DT, Liotta AS, Suda T, Goodgold A, Condon E (1979) Human plasma immunoreactive lipotropin and ACTH in normal subjects and in patients with pituitary-adrenal disease. J Clin Endocrinol Metab 48:566–571

Krieger DT, Luria M (1977) Plasma ACTH and cortisol responses to TRF, vasopressin and hypoglycemia in Cushing's disease and Nelson's syndrome. J Clin Endocrinol Metab 44:361–368

Krieger DT, Samojlik E, Bardin CW (1978) Cortisol and androgen secretion in a case of Nelson's syndrome with paratesticular tumors: Response to cyproheptadine therapy. J Clin Endocrinol Metab 47:837–844

Laidlaw JC, Jenkins D, Reddy WJ, Harrison JH, Thorn GW (1954) Diagnosis of hyperadrenocorticism. J Clin Endocrinol Metab 14:781 (Abstract)

Lamberts SWJ, deJong FH, Birkenhager JC (1977) Evaluation of diagnostic and differential diagnostic tests in Cushing's syndrome. Neth J Med 20:267–274

Leach RB, Margulis RR (1965) Inhibition of adrenocortical responsiveness during progestin therapy. Am J Obstet Gynecol 92:762–765

Lecky MW, Wolfman NT, Modic CW (1976) Current concepts of adrenal angiography. Radiol Clin North Am 14:209–252

Liddle GW (1960) Tests of pituitary-adrenal suppressibility in the diagnosis of Cushing's syndrome. J Clin Endocrinol Metab 20:1539–1559

Liddle GW, Estep HL, Kendall JW Jr, Williams WC Jr, Townes AW (1959) Clinical application of a new test of pituitary reserve. J Clin Endocrinol Metab 19:875–894

Liddle GW, Melmon KL (1974) The adrenals. In: Williams RH (ed) Textbook of endocrinology, 5th ed. Saunders, Philadelphia, pp 233–322

Lieberman LM, Beierwaltes WH, Conn JW, Ansari AN, Nishiyams H (1971) Diagnosis of adrenal disease by visualization of human adrenal glands with $^{131}$I-19-iodocholesterol. N Engl J Med 285:1387–1393
Linn JE Jr, Bowdoin B, Farmer TA, Meador CK (1967) Observations and comments on failure of dexamethasone suppression. N Engl J Med 277:403–405
Lipscomb H, Nelson DM (1962) A sensitive biological assay for ACTH. Endocrinology 71:13–23
Ludecke D, Kautzky R, Saeger W, Schrader D (1976) Selective removal of hypersecreting adenomas? An analysis of endocrine function, operative and microscopical findings in 101 cases. Acta Neurochir (Wien) 35:27–42
Luton JP, Thieblot P, Valcke C, Mahoudea JA, Bricaire H (1977) Reversible gonadotropin deficiency in male Cushing's disease. J Clin Endocrinol Metab 45:488–495
MacErlean DP, Doyle FH (1976) The pituitary fossa in Cushing's syndrome: A retrospective analysis of 93 patients. Br J Radiol 49:820–826
McKenna TJ, Lorber D, Lacroix A, Rabin D (1979) Testicular activity in Cushing's disease. Acta Endocrinol 91:501–510
Meikle AW, Lagerquist LG, Tyler FH (1975) Apparently normal pituitary-adrenal suppressibility in Cushing's syndrome: Dexamethasone metabolism and plasma levels. J Lab Clin Med 86:472–478
Meikle AW, Stanchfield JB, West CD, Tyler FH (1974) Hydrocortisone suppression test for Cushing's syndrome: Therapy with anticonvulsants. Arch Intern Med 134:1068–1071
Miles JM, Wahner HW, Carpenter PC, Salassa RM, Northcutt RC (1979) Adrenal scintiscanning with NP-59, a new radioiodinated cholesterol agent. Mayo Clin Proc 54:321–327
Mitty HA, Nicolis GL, Gabrilove JL (1973) Adrenal venography: Clinical-roentgenographic correlation in 80 patients. Am J Roentgenol 129:564–575
Nichols T, Nugent CA, Tyler FH (1968) Steroid laboratory tests in the diagnosis of Cushing's syndrome. Am J Med 45:116–128
Nugent CA, MacDiarmid WD, Nelson AR, Tyler FH (1963) Rate of adrenal cortisol production in response to maximal stimulation with ACTH. J Clin Endocrinol Metab 23:684–693
Nugent CA, Nichols T, Tyler FH (1965) Diagnosis of Cushing's syndrome: Single-dose dexamethasone suppression test. Arch Intern Med 116:172–176
Oki S, Nakai Y, Nakao K, Imura H (1980) Plasma $\beta$-endorphin responses to somatostatin, thyrotropin-releasing hormone, or vasopressin in Nelson's syndrome. J Clin Endocrinol Metab 50:194–197
Olsen NJ, Fang VS, DeGroot LJ (1978) Cushing's syndrome due to adrenal adenoma with persistent diurnal cortisol secretory rhythm. Metabolism 27:695–700
Pavlatos FC, Smilo RP, Forsham PH (1965) A rapid screening test for Cushing's syndrome. JAMA 193:720–723
Pieters GFFM, Smals, AGH, Benraad TJ, Kloppenborg PWC (1979) Plasma cortisol response to thyrotropin-releasing hormone and luteinizing hormone-releasing hormone in Cushing's disease. J Clin Endocrinol Metab 48:874–876
Porter CC, Silber RH (1950) A quantitative color reaction for cortisone and related 17,21-dihydroxy-20-ketosteroids. J Biol Chem 185:201–207
Raux MC, Binoux M, Luton JP, Gourmelin M, Girard F (1975) Studies of ACTH secretion control in 116 cases of Cushing's syndrome. J Clin Endocrinol Metab 40:186–197
Rayfield EJ, Rose LI, Cain JP, Dluhy RG, Williams GH (1971) ACTH-responsive, dexamethasone-suppressible adrenocortical carcinoma. N Engl J Med 284:591–592
Rees LH, Romlin SJ, Ratter SJ, Jeffcoate WJ, Nichol W (1978) ACTH/lipotropin (LPH) measurements in the localization of ectopic ACTH-secreting tumours. 60th Meeting. Endocrin. Soc., p 197
Rivarola MA, Saez JM, Meyers WJ, Jenkins ME, Migeon CJ (1966) Metabolic clearance rate and blood production rate of testosterone and androst-4-ene 3, 17-dione under basal conditions, ACTH and hCG stimulation: Comparison with urinary production rate of testosterone. J Clin Endocrinol Metab 26:1208–1218
Rovit RL, Duane TD (1969) Cushing's syndrome and pituitary tumors: Pathophysiology and ocular manifestations of ACTH-secreting pituitary adenomas. Am J Med 46:416–427
Sakar SD, Cohen EL, Beierwaltes WH, Ice RD, Cooper R, Gold EN (1977) A new and superior adrenal imaging agent, $^{131}$I-6$\beta$-iodomethyl-19-nor-cholesterol (NP-59): Evaluation in humans. J Clin Endocrinol Metab 45:353–362

Salassa RM, Kearns TP, Hernohan JW, Sprague RG, MacCarty CS (1959) Pituitary tumors in patients with Cushing's syndrome. J Clin Endocrinol Metab 19:1523–1539
Salassa RM, Laws ER Jr, Carpenter PC, Northcutt RC (1978) Transsphenoidal removal of pituitary microadenoma in Cushing's disease. Mayo Clin Proc 53:24–28
Schambelan M, Slaton PE Jr, Biglieri EG (1971) Mineralocorticoid production in hyperadrenocorticism: Role in pathogenesis of hypokalemia alkalosis. Am J Med 51:299–303
Schteingart DE, Conn JW, Lieberman LM, Beierwaltes WJ (1972) Persistent or recurrent Cushing's syndrome after "total" adrenalectomy. Arch Intern Med 130:384–387
Seabold JE, Bernardino ME, Goldstein HM, Green B, Glenn HJ, Haynie TP (1978) Comparison of adrenal scintigraphy, ultrasonography and computerized tomography in the evaluation of suspected adrenal lesions (abstract). Int J Nucl Med Biol 5:202–203
Sederberg-Olsen P, Binder C, Kehlet H, Neville AM, Nielsen LM (1973) Episodic variation in plasma corticosteroids in subjects with Cushing's syndrome of differing etiology. J Clin Endocrinol Metab 36:906–910
Silverman SR, Marnell RT, Sholiton LJ, Werk EE Jr (1963) Failure of dexamethasone suppression test to indicate bilateral adrenocortical hyperplasia in Cushing's syndrome. J Clin Endocrinol Metab 23:167–172
Smals AGH, Kloppenborg PWC, Benraad TJ (1977) Plasma testosterone profiles in Cushing's syndrome. J Clin Endocrinol Metab 45:240–245
Spiger M, Jubiz W, Meikle AW, West CD, Tyler FH (1975) Single-dose metyrapone test. Arch Intern Med 135:698–700
Staub JJ, Girard J, Noelpp B, Baumann JB, Graf S, Ratcliffe JG (1979) The short metyrapone test: Comparison of the plasma ACTH response to metyrapone and insulin-induced hypoglycaemia. Clin Endocrinol 10:595–602
Streeten DHP, Stevenson CT, Dalakos TG, Nicholas JJ, Dennick LG, Fellerman H (1969) The diagnosis of hypercortisolism. Biochemical criteria differentiating patients from lean and obese normal subjects and from females on oral contraceptives. J Clin Endocrinol Metab 29:1191–1211
Suda T, Liotta AS, Krieger DT (1978) β-Endorphin is not detectable in plasma from normal subjects. Science 202:221–223
Swanson HA, du Boulay G (1975) Borderline variants of the normal pituitary fossa. Br J Radiol 48:366–369
Tyrrell JB, Brooks RM, Fitzgerald PA, Cofoid PB, Forsham PH, Wilson CB (1978) Cushing's disease: Selective trans-sphenoidal resection of pituitary microadenomas. N Engl J Med 298:753–758
Tyrrell JB, Lorenzi M, Forsham PH, Gerich JE (1975) The effect of somatostatin on secretion of adrenocorticotropin in normal subjects and in patients with Nelson's syndrome and Cushing's disease. 57th Meeting Endocrin. Soc., p 350
Tyrrell JB, Wiener-Kronish J, Lorenzi M, Brooks RM, Forsham PH (1977) Cushing's disease: Growth hormone response to hypoglycemia after correction of hypercortisolism J Clin Endocrinol Metab 44:218–221
Vagnucci AH (1979) Analysis of circadian periodicity of plasma cortisol in normal man and in Cushing's syndrome. Am J Physiol 236:R268–R281
Van Cauter E, Huyberechts R (1973) Problems in the statistical analysis of biological time series: The cosinor test and the periodogram. J Interdiscip Cycle Res 4:41–57
Van Cauter EV, Leclercq R, Vanhaelst L, Golstein J (1974) Simultaneous study of cortisol and TSH daily variations in normal subjects and patients with hyperadrenalcorticism. J Clin Endocrinol Metab 39:645–652
Weinstein M, Tyrrell B, Newton TH (1976) The sella turcica in Nelson's syndrome. Radiology 118:363–365
Welbourn RB, Montgomery DAD, Kennedy TL (1971) The natural history of treated Cushing's syndrome. Br J Surg 58:1–16
West CD, Dolman LI (1977) Plasma ACTH radioimmunoassays in the diagnosis of pituitary-adrenal dysfunction. In: Krieger DT, Ganong WF (eds) ACTH and related peptides: Structure, regulation and action. N.Y. Acad. Sci., New York, pp 205–217
West CD, Meikle AW (1979) Laboratory tests for the diagnosis of Cushing's syndrome in adrenal insufficiency and factors affecting those tests. In: DeGroot LJ et al. (eds) Endocrinology, vol. 2. Grune and Stratton, New York

West CD, Meikle AW, Ganguly A, Stanchfield JB, Atcheson JB, Tyler FH (1979) Multiple steroid abnormalities in Cushing's syndrome. 61st Meeting Endocrin. Soc., p 235
Wiedemann E, Saito T, Linfoot JA (1978) Independent regulation of plasma beta-lipotropin and ACTH in patients with Cushing's disease and acromegaly (abstract). Clin Res 26:108A
Yalow RS, Berson SA (1973) Characteristics of "big ACTH" in human plasma and pituitary extracts. J Clin Endocrinol Metab 36:415–423
Yalow RS, Glick SM, Roth J, Berson SA (1964) Radioimmunoassay of human plasma ACTH. J Clin Endocrinol Metab 24:1219–1225
Yamaguchi H, Liotta AS, Krieger DT (1980) Simultaneous determination of human plasma immunoreactive β-lipotropin, γ-lipotropin, and β-endorphin utilizing immune-affinity chromatography. J Clin Endocrinol Metab 51:1002–1008
Yeh H-C, Mitty HA, Rose J, Wolf BS, Gabrilove JL (1978) Ultrasonography of adrenal masses: Usual features. Radiology 127:467–474
Yoshida K, Satowa H, Sato A, Ichikawa Y, Kream J, Levin J, Zumoff B, Hellman L, Fukushima DK (1979) Plasma cortisol profiles in Cushing's syndrome. Acta Endocrinol 91:319–328
Zimmerman CE, Eisenberg H, Spark R, Rosoff CB (1974) Transvenous adrenal destruction: Clinical trials in patients with metastatic malignancy. Surgery 75:550–556
Zumoff B, Fukushima DK, Weitzman ED, Kream J, Hellman L (1974) The sex difference in plasma cortisol concentration in man. J Clin Endocrinol Metab 39:805–808

*Chapter 8*

# Treatment of Cushing's Disease and Syndrome

## A. Adrenal Adenoma

Cure can be achieved by adrenal extirpation. This is performed by a flank approach, since such tumors are almost always unilateral. Because of the associated atrophy of the contralateral adrenal, patients will require postoperative replacement therapy for a variable time period (3–18 months) until normal adrenocortical function is regained. Cortisol replacement therapy should be maintained at a sufficient dose to avoid symptoms of hypoadrenalism without being so excessive as to prevent recovery of the suppressed pituitary ACTH secretion, which is secondary to the prior hypercortisolism produced by the adenoma. There is no evidence that ACTH treatment to enhance adrenal responsiveness will hasten recovery of such suppressed function, since recovery at the pituitary level takes a longer time than does that of adrenal responsiveness to ACTH, and the excess cortisol secretion engendered by such ACTH administration might further delay pituitary recovery.

## B. Adrenocortical Carcinoma

Since at diagnosis these tumors show local spread in approximately 65% of cases (Hutter and Kayhoe 1966), surgical cure is uncommon. In the series reported by Lipsett et al. (1963), attempted local curative excision could be performed in only 18 of 38 cases. Even with such attempted local excision, only 7 of the 18 were alive after a 5-year period. When curative resection was not performed, 70% of the patients died within 2 years. There is a report that the survival time in untreated patients is 2.9 months following diagnosis (MacFarlane 1958). Therefore, in those patients in whom attempted resection is performed, as well as in those in whom resection cannot be performed because of local invasion and/or metastases, drug therapy to inhibit adrenal steroid biosynthesis may offer symptomatic relief from the metabolic consequences of hypercorticism. The two drugs most frequently employed in the treatment of adrenal carcinoma are o,p′DDD and aminoglutethimide.

### I. o,p′DDD (Lysodren, Mitotane)

Following the observation that administration of the insecticide DDD to dogs resulted in necrosis and atrophy of the adrenal cortex, it was found that the o,p′DDD isomer had markedly enhanced activity as compared to the crude DDD. Necrosis and atrophy were specific for the zona reticularis and the zona fasciculata. It was also observed that this drug blocked corticosteroidogenesis by a variety of enzymatic mechanisms. o,p'DDD (Lysodren; Mitotane) has, therefore, been employed in the treatment of both functioning and nonfunctioning adrenal carcinoma over the past 20 years. The maximum dose tolerated by most adults with minimal side effects is 10 g daily. Side effects include gastrointestinal upset, which may be ameliorated by temporary reduction of dosage; CNS effects, i.e., somnolence, which can also be reversed with reduction of dosage; and rashes, which will disappear without discontinuance of therapy.

In both functioning and nonfunctioning tumors, documented regression of adrenal masses and metastatic lesions has been reported in approximately 40%–60% of the cases (Hutter and Kayhoe 1966; Lubitz et al. 1973). Hormonal responses are seen in approximately 70% of patients with functioning tumors. However, since o,p'DDD alters the extra-adrenal metabolism of cortisol, 17-OHCS measurements should be followed by determinations of urinary or plasma cortisol. Positive hormonal responses are evident in most patients within 30 days after initiation of therapy, with a mean duration of response of approximately 10 months. Steroid responses occurred in all patients showing an objective tumor response. The converse, however, is not necessarily so. In view of the relatively small number of patients so treated, it is not possible to determine whether an actual statistical increase in survival has been accomplished, although this appears to be the case. There have been two reports of apparent long-term cures (Becker and Schumacher 1975; Ostuni and Roginsky 1975).

### II. Aminoglutethimide

This drug is available only for investigative purposes. Approximately 60% of patients show both clinical and biochemical improvement, but not all biochemical responses are accompanied by a tumoricidal effect. A dose of 1–2 g daily is usually employed. The most common toxic manifestations are somnolence, which may be mild and transient, and rash, which will disappear spontaneously when drug therapy is continued. No long-term responses have been reported and there are no adequate data with regard to mean duration of therapeutic response, which appears to be shorter than that noted for o,p'DDD (Misbin et al. 1976).

## C. Ectopic ACTH-Producing Tumors

If tumor resection can be performed and no metastases are present, cure may be achieved. Such instances are most likely in cases of bronchial carcinoid, thymoma, and medullary thyroid carcinoma. In cases with metastatic lesions for which there is effective chemotherapy, such therapy may also suppress the hormonal activity of the tumor (Walter et al. 1973; Rees et al. 1977). In those patients in whom survival expectancy is more than a matter of months, some clinical amelioration may be accomplished by the use of adrenolytic agents, such as o,p'DDD, aminoglutethimide, or metyrapone, to bring about symptomatic relief from the concomitant hypercortisolism.

## D. Cushing's Disease

There are rare cases of Cushing's disease (as noted in Chap. 6, p 52) in which spontaneous remissions have been described. There are also reports of cases (i. e., Minnie, one of Cushing's original cases) with a prolonged, but not incapacitating clinical course without therapeutic intervention. From available data it would appear, however, that with no treatment approximately 50% of patients with Cushing's disease will succumb within 5 years of diagnosis. The major causes of death are infection (even with concomitant antibiotic therapy) and complications from generalized arteriosclerosis, such as cardiac failure, myocardial infarction, and cerebrovascular accidents (Plotz et al. 1952). It is within this framework that one can begin to evaluate the therapeutic efficacy of the various regimens proposed since Cushing's initial description of this disease.

The ideal objective of treatment is to correct the cause by permanently removing the stimulus for increased cortisol production, which is responsible for most of the clinical manifestations. All of the suggested forms of therapy should ideally correct the hypercortisolism without introducing other associated endocrine deficiencies (i. e., adrenal or pituitary insufficiency). Since, as discussed in previous chapters, the etiology of Cushing's disease is not fully understood, various available therapies have been directed either at correction of the enhanced cortisol secretion, through either surgical or medical adrenalectomy, or to reduce or remove the enhanced secretion of ACTH. This may be accomplished by pituitary irradiation or by surgical removal of the pituitary macro- or microadenomas. Recently, as a result of neuropharmacological studies on the regulation of CRF and ACTH release and evidence indicating altered CNS regulation of pituitary function in Cushing's disease, attempts at neuropharmacological therapy have also been reported.

Figure 8.1 indicates the hierarchy of CNS-pituitary-adrenocortical regulation, as well as the points at which the various therapeutic measures have been postulated to act. Pituitary irradiation is presumed to act directly on the pituitary although, in view of the greater radiosensitivity of the hypothalamus than the pituitary, the question has been raised as to whether the major effect may be on the former. It is apparent that when local pituitary implantation of radioactive substances is performed this effect would be a direct pituitary one. Neuropharmacological agents commonly employed are believed to act via alterations in neural pathways regulating various aspects of CRF release, although there has been some question as to a possible direct pituitary effect of cyproheptadine when employed as an antiserotonergic agent (see below). Although the various adrenolytic agents employed have all been demonstrated to have direct effects on enzymatic steps involved in steroidogenesis, there is also some evidence that metyrapone may act directly on the pituitary gland.

All of these forms of therapy have succeeded in correcting hypercortisolism, successfully treated patients with Cushing's disease being no more at risk of decreased longevity than those without the disease, except for possible effects of pre-existing atherosclerosis. In addition to its inherent efficacy, the choice of a given therapy may also be influenced by the need for rapid control of

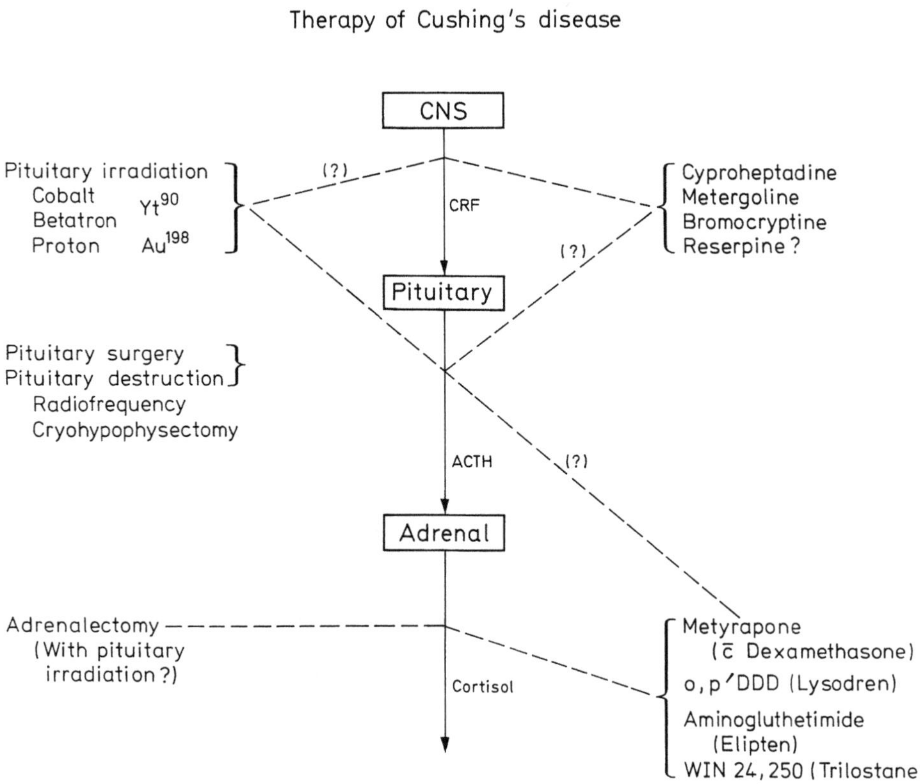


**Fig. 8.1.** Locus of action of therapy employed in the treatment of Cushing's disease

the hypercortisolemic state and its complications. Manifestations that require rapid reversal of hypercortisolism include progressive hypertension, severe and progressive osteoporosis, and psychiatric disturbances. In such instances, therapeutic approaches that may require a moderately prolonged time period before maximum therapeutic effect is observed, such as pituitary irradiation and some forms of medical therapy, would be less desirable than surgical approaches preferably directed at the pituitary.

## I. Adrenal Surgery

Following Cushing's initial report of the disease, some early therapeutic failures following pituitary irradiation led to the approach of surgical resection of the adrenals. These early procedures are well summarized by Cope and Raker (1955), who advocated subtotal resection similar to what had been successfully used in the surgical treatment of Graves' disease. It became evident that greater than 90% resection was probably required, and it came to be appreciated that those subjects in whom a good therapeutic response was obtained could not be weaned away from the postoperative cortisone replacement and thus remained permanently adrenal insufficient. If such weaning could be accomplished, it usually signified future recurrence (Welbourn et al. 1971). There have been several recent series summarizing the effects of total bilateral adrenalectomy (Ernest and Ekman 1972; Bennett et al. 1973; Scott et al. 1977). It is now generally agreed that a bilateral flank approach is associated with less operative morbidity and mortality than the transabdominal approach previously advocated. An operative mortality varying from 5%–10% has been reported, usually from embolic phenomena (which may be aggravated by the hypercortisolemic state), as well as complications from wound infection and postoperative bleeding. (In the future, it may well be that attempts at reduction of hypercortisolemia by medical means prior to adrenalectomy will prevent those surgical complications associated with the hypercortisolemic state at the time of surgery.) There have also been several deaths during the 1st year postoperative period that may be attributed to established concomitants of the disease prior to surgery, such as cardiac or cerebrovascular disease. Five to ten percent of cases may show evidence of persistent cortisol secretion postoperatively, despite total adrenalectomy, because of the presence of adrenocortical remnants. Detection and removal of such remnants represents a formidable problem.

Parenteral hydrocortisone administration (usually amounting to 300 mg daily) begins the day of surgery, with a decrease to maintenance requirements (parenterally or orally) over the ensuing week. It should be realized that the exact mode and time course of such a decrease will be governed by the patient's postoperative course. Patients usually require daily maintenance of 25–37.5 mg cortisone acetate or 20–30 mg hydrocortisone daily, with two-thirds of the dose being given in the morning and the remainder in the late afternoon. Mineralocorticoid replacement may or may not be required. Adequacy of maintenance dosage can be followed by determining plasma cortisol concentrations 30–60 min after a given dose. Patients should be instructed as to the risk during stressful situations, such as febrile illnesses, acute gastrointestinal infections, and incidental surgical procedures. It is advisable to provide them with a kit with facilities for parenteral steroid administration, as well as a Medicalert bracelet identifying them as adrenalectomized individuals.

In female subjects, menses usually return within 7 months postoperatively. The diabetic state usually improves. Body weight returns to normal in two-thirds of the patients, although in the remainder there may still be evidence of a cushingoid facial habitus with normal adrenocortical steroid concentrations. The pain associated with osteoporosis usually disappears, although there is no reversal of the osteoporosis except in very young subjects. In most patients, mental changes are markedly improved, although in a small minority these may persist and be responsible for some additional postoperative morbidity and mortality. Half of the patients with preexisting hypertension, although exhibiting some decrease, may still have moderately elevated blood pressure levels. Lastly, the development of Nelson's syndrome in 15%–20% of the bilaterally adrenalectomized patients has already been discussed. It had been thought that by combining adrenalectomy with pituitary irradiation the incidence of this complication would be lessened, but available data indicate that this does not appear to be the case.

The necessity for continued corticosteroid replacement has tempted some surgeons over the last decade to consider combining total adrenalectomy with autotransplantation of part of the adrenals. There are isolated reports of success and failure of such procedures (Prinz et al. 1979; Barzilai et al. 1980). Even in the case reported by Prinz et al., in whom remission has been maintained for 11 years following surgery, plasma ACTH concentrations remain moderately elevated (167–230 pg/ml) and, as expected, only partial suppression of plasma cortisol was present in response to overnight dexamethasone administration. With the recent advent of radionuclide scanning, visualization of such adrenal transplants can be performed to demonstrate graft function and to indicate the appropriate time of weaning such patients from corticosteroid therapy.

It appears, therefore, that bilateral adrenalectomy should be reserved at present only for those cases in whom other therapeutic approaches have failed. In conditions where rapid reversal of the hypercortisolemic state is required, the removal of a pituitary tumor or microadenoma can accomplish this without the added difficulty of permanent adrenocortical insufficiency.

### II. Adrenal-Directed Pharmacological Therapy

Four drugs are available that act by inhibition of steroidogenesis.

The drug o,p'DDD (Mitotane, Lysodren) has already been discussed with regard to its use in the treatment of adrenal carcinoma. The most extensive report of its use in treatment of Cushing's disease is by Luton et al. (1979). Of patients treated over an 8-month period with doses of 6–12 g daily, 82% showed initial response; however, more than 50% of these patients subsequently relapsed, requiring further treatment. Subsequent additional courses of therapy combined with pituitary irradiation resulted in an overall remission rate of 60%. Noted side effects included increased serum cholesterol and alkaline phosphatase concentrations (not associated with other evidence of hepatic dysfunction), as well as symptoms of mineralocorticoid insufficiency, in contrast to the reported absence of the latter effects in the series of Orth and Liddle (1971). There were no other significant side effects unlike previous studies (see "Adrenocortical Carcinoma"); the authors attributed this to their use of capsules in which the drug was mixed with cellulose acetylphthalate. Orth and Liddle (1971) reported cures in all of eight patients treated with 3–6 g daily over a 4–6-month period, and subsequent smaller maintenance doses. Most of the patients experienced a major loss of adrenocortical reserve with such treatment, requiring maintenance corticosteroid therapy. That this may be a necessary concomitant of effective therapy is suggested by Luton et al. (1979): a relapse could be predicted when adrenal insufficiency was not obtained (although relapse could be seen even when such insufficiency occurred) or when adrenal glands were still detectable on $^{131}$I-iodocholesterol scan. Effective lowering of corticosteroid concentrations to the normal range may take as long as 4–6 months following initiation of therapy.

Aminoglutethimide (Elipten) has also been discussed with regard to its use in adrenocortical carcinoma. The drug is available only for investigative use. Although, based upon effects on inhibition of steroidogenesis (by interference with conversion of cholesterol to pregnenolone) in addition to blocking various steroid hydroxylations, the drug might be expected to interfere with ovarian and testicular steroidogenesis, such effects have not been studied in patients with Cushing's disease receiving relatively long-term treatment. Unlike o,p'DDD therapy, with which several months are required before suppression of adrenal secretion is seen, frank adrenal insufficiency may appear within 5 days following onset of aminoglutethimide therapy. Its efficiency in Cushing's disease (where adrenal secretion is ACTH dependent), unlike in adrenal carcinoma (where secretion is ACTH independent), appears to be limited, since drug escape with resumption of enhanced steroidogenesis usually occurs as the result of compensatory increases in ACTH secretion sufficient to break through the initially effective enzymatic blockade. Fishman et al. (1967), however, reported continued responsiveness in two of three patients receiving treatment over a 6-month period. Misbin et al. (1976) report an overall, relatively short clinical and biochemical improvement in 42% of treated patients. Side effects, such as goiter, somnolence, and skin rashes, have been reported with the usual therapeutic doses of 0.75–1.5 g/day, such symptoms disappearing with drug discontinuance. Combined use of aminoglutethimide and metyrapone (see below) has been advocated, with reports of reduced toxicity as the result of employment of lower doses of each of these compounds.

Metyrapone is effective in lowering cortisol production by inhibition both of 11-$\beta$-hydroxylation and of cholesterol cleavage to pregnenolone. In view of the observation that some patients receiving this medication for long-term management of Cushing's disease exhibited a decrease in plasma ACTH concentrations following long-term treatment, this has led to the suggestion that a direct, perhaps paradoxical effect on the pituitary also existed, although this may well have been the effect of the concurrent pituitary irradiation received by such patients (Jeffcoate et al. 1977). Responses with regard to normalization of urinary corticosteroid excretion were usually rapid and the expected "overshoot" of plasma ACTH levels was not noted. In this report total duration of treatment was 21 months, with the duration of follow-up unclear. Few side effects were noted, except for increasing hirsutism in some patients. In view of the 11-$\beta$-hydroxylase block, the drug might be contraindicated in patients with marked hypertension because of the concomitant increases in mineralocorticoid concentrations secondary to such 11-$\beta$-hydroxylase blockade. As noted above, metyrapone has been combined with aminoglutethimide, as well as with dexamethasone and fluorocortisone (to suppress any possible rise in plasma ACTH concentrations resulting from decreased adrenal cortisol secretion), with favorable rapid responses in five patients and with persisting efficacy in long-term treatment (varying from 30 to 365 days in three of four patients) (Child et al. 1976).

Metyrapone and aminoglutethimide, singly or in combination, are best utilized not as primary therapy for normalizing adrenocortical function, but in preparing patients for surgery or while awaiting achievement of a therapeutic response to pituitary irradiation. Since adrenal insufficiency may be seen with the use of these agents, concomitant dexamethasone administration is usually indicated.

Trilostane has been employed in one investigational study in which clinical and laboratory improvement were reported in all of seven patients without any significant treatment-related side effects (Komanicky et al. 1978). Only two of the patients received therapy for more than 1 month. The drug acts as an inhibitor of the $3\beta$-HSDH-$\Delta^{4-5}$ isomerase enzyme system. Escape may also occur because of associated secondary rises in ACTH secretion.

## III. Pituitary Irradiation

Pituitary irradiation can be accomplished by conventional cobalt radiotherapy (approximately 4500 rad), by proton beam irradiation, or by pituitary implantation of radioactive material. There is still disagreement as to the efficacy of conventional radiotherapy. A survey of the literature (Table 8.1) (Dohan et al. 1957; Soffer et al. 1961; Heuschele and Lampe 1967; Orth and Liddle 1971; van Seters et al. 1975) indicated that 46%–83% of the patients are improved. Within each reported series, approximately two-thirds of the responses noted are cures, with the remainder representing significant improvement with only modest elevations of corticosteroid concentrations and minimal disability. The major disadvantage of such therapy is the prolonged time necessary for improvement to occur, which may be as long as 18 months following completion of radiotherapy, although a response is usually seen within the 1st year. Because of this, it is usually suggested that patients be treated with concomitant pituitary or adrenal suppression therapy if feasible. o,p'DDD would be less preferable than the other agents available, since with this drug permanent adrenal atrophy may occur.

Pituitary irradiation is a procedure that is virtually free of morbidity and does not occasion any other endocrine deficits. There is no evidence of pituitary dysfunction with regard to other pituitary hormones following such therapy. Indeed, there is restoration of normal fertility in adults, and no effect on subsequent fertility as well as restoration of normal growth rates in children with the disease. In children, pituitary irradiation may be even more efficacious than in adults. Jennings et al. (1977) reported cure of 12 of 15 children utilizing doses ranging from 3500 to 4950 rad. Growth resumed and sexual development proceeded normally in all. The age at treatment was 8–16 years, with follow-up periods of 1–18 years. There was no evidence of any subsequent progressive pituitary enlargement.

**Table 8.1.** Cushing's disease: Effect of pituitary irradiation

| | N | Improved (%) |
|---|---|---|
| Cobalt | 100 | 46–83[a] |
| Au 198 or Y 90 | 57 | 66–71[a] |
| Proton | 21 (1969)[c] | 64–80[b] |
| | ca. 105 (1979)[c] | 89–95 |

[a] Cure or persistence of only moderate disease.
[b] Cure.
[c] Date of report.

Pituitary implantation of radioactive gold or yttrium has been the subject of investigation by a group of English investigators (Burke et al. 1972). The X-ray appearance of the fossa appears to be an important factor in predicting outcome. Eighty-one percent of patients improved who showed no evidence of pituitary tumor on routine sellar X-rays while only 50% showed improvement when there were minor abnormalities of size or shape on routine sellar X-rays, which were confirmed on tomography. When there was definite X-ray evidence of pituitary tumor, only 15% of patients showed improvement. This form of therapy requires a short period of hospitalization. The median interval between implantation and demonstration of complete remission is approximately 4 months. The complication of cerebrospinal fluid (CSF) rhinorrhea has decreased since this form of therapy was first introduced. Steroid replacement therapy is required in approximately half of the patients.

Heavy-particle radiation has been employed by two groups, Linfoot (1979) and Kjellberg and Kliman (1973). By utilization of the Bragg peak effect, doses as high as 15000 rad may be delivered to the center of the pituitary, with a decrease at a rate of 1000–2000 rad/min. Accurate dosage requires an exact estimate of pituitary dimensions in cases where there is no obvious tumor. Computerized tomography and cavernous sinography are necessary to delineate superior and lateral extension in cases with gross evidence of tumor. A cure rate of approximately 90%–95% is reported, with, however, an incidence of partial or panhypopituitrism of 7%–10%. There may be neurophthalmological deficits after treatment, which are usually transient. Unlike other methods of pituitary irradiation where a low percentage of relapse may occur, no instances of relapse have been reported following heavy-particle irradiation.

### IV. Pituitary Surgery

Prior to the last decade, pituitary surgery for Cushing's disease was performed only in instances where gross pituitary tumors were demonstrated. With the advent of transsphenoidal microsurgery, the recent interest in pituitary polytomography, the demonstration of other functional microadenomas (especially prolactinomas), and the known incidence of such microadenomas in patients with Cushing's disease (see Chap. 6), there has been a reawakening of interest in management of Cushing's disease by transsphenoidal pituitary microsurgery. There have been four large series reported in which microadenectomy was performed, comprised of 85 patients (Salassa et al. 1978; Tyrrell et al. 1978; Bigos et al. 1980; Kuwayama et al. 1980), as well as other series (Ludecke et al. 1976; Carmalt et al. 1977) in which complete or partial hypophysectomy was performed. Although data are limited, it appears that those cases where there is localized invasion coupled with or without suprasellar extension have a less favorable response than when such tumors are localized entirely within the pituitary (Fig. 8.2).

From these reports, it is also apparent that microadenomas will be found irrespective of whether tomography is associated with positive findings. For example, although surgery was performed only in those 18 patients with positive X-ray findings in the series reported by Salassa et al. (1978), adenomas were found in 17. In the series reported by Tyrrell et al. (1978), of eight

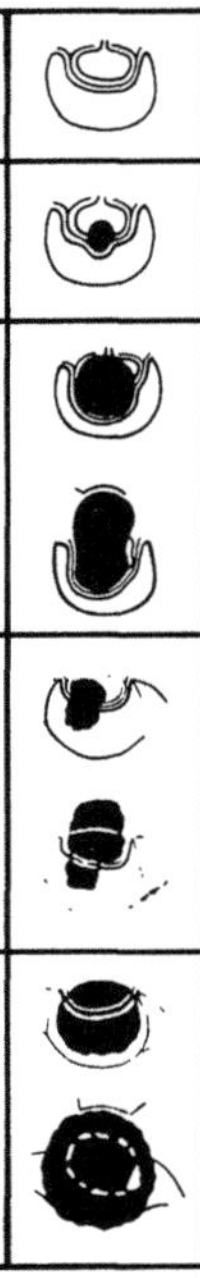

| SELLA TURCICA RADIOLOGICAL CLASSIFICATION | | | | NO. OF CASES | CURED |
|---|---|---|---|---|---|
| ADENOMAS | ENCLOSED | GRADE 0 | NORMAL | 10 | 8 |
| | | GRADE I <10 mm | MICRO-ADENOMA | 8 | 7 |
| | | GRADE II >10 mm | NO SSE | 3 | 3 |
| | | | SSE | | |
| | INVASIVES | GRADE III LOCALIZED | NO SSE | 2 | 0 |
| | | | SSE | | |
| | | GRADE IV DIFFUSE | NO SSE | 1 | 0 |
| | | | SSE | | |
| TOTAL | | | | 24 | 18 |

**Fig. 8.2.** Efficacy of transphenoidal surgery for Cushing's disease classified according to nature of pituitary pathology. *SSE* indicates suprasellar extension. From Bigos et al. (1980) with permission

patients with normal sellar tomograms who were explored, five had intrasellar abnormalities; in one no intrasellar abnormality was located, but a 1.5 mm basophilic adenoma was found in the specimen removed by total hypophysectomy. In two others, technical failure precluded surgical correction, and no specimen was obtained. In the series reported by Bigos et al. (1980), normal sellar tomography was present in 10 of 24 patients; in seven of these with normal tomography, microadenomata were found.

The surgical cure rate reported varies from 85% in the series of Tyrrell et al. (1978) (90% if the case with total hypophysectomy is included), with 6-month follow-up; 70% in the series of Salassa et al. (1978), in whom 13 of the 18 cases were followed up for more than 2 years; and 66% in the series of Bigos et al. (1980) (if one includes all operated cases, or 76% if one excludes cases where tumors were characterized as invasive). The duration of follow-up in this series was 1–180 months, with a median follow-up of 12 months.

Complications related to surgery were present in approximately 7% of patients, including bleeding or CSF rhinorrhea. A small percentage also developed transient diabetes insipidus. In the series reported by Bigos et al., two recurrences were evident after 10 and 30 months of remission (see below).

Exploration of one revealed a normal pituitary, with cure by total hypophysectomy. In the other patient, cure was effected by pituitary irradiation. In the series of Salassa et al., 2 of the 18 patients had persisting disease postoperatively, in one of whom an adenoma had been removed, while in the other there had been no surgical evidence of adenoma, and no definite tumor could be identified by posmortem examination of the pituitary.

Postoperative studies of these patients have revealed several interesting findings. Tyrrell et al. (1978) reported markedly reduced postoperative plasma ACTH levels and plasma and urinary corticosteroid concentrations in all patients throughout the 6 months of postoperative observation. In the series reported by Bigos et al. (1980), however, only 3 of 16 patients required postoperative corticoid replacement therapy. Tyrrell's patients had been maintained on replacement hydrocortisone (20–30 mg/day) throughout this period, a dose considered insufficient in itself to cause sustained suppression of ACTH and adrenocortical secretion in patients with Cushing's disease. The patients also exhibited decreased responsiveness of plasma ACTH and corticosteroids to insulin-induced hypoglycemia (Fitzgerald et al. 1978), with some improvement, although not to the normal range, when studied 12 months postoperatively. (The nature of steroid replacement at the time of the last study was not given and data are not available from individual patients.) Kuwayama et al. (1980) have noted postoperative adrenal insufficiency, decreased responsiveness of plasma ACTH concentrations to lysine vasopressin administration, but normal responses to insulin-induced hypoglycemia. In one case studied by Lagerquist et al. (1974), no response to insulin-induced hypoglycemia was present at 8 months, with no report of testing earlier in the postoperative period. These discrepancies make it somewhat difficult to ascertain whether the locus of postoperative suppression is at the CNS or pituitary level. Interpretation is also somewhat clouded when studies are performed using physiological or slightly more than physiological corticosteroid replacement.

Other studies have evaluated the return of normal dexamethasone suppressibility and circadian corticosteroid periodicity. Schnall et al. (1978) noted return of normal circadian periodicity at 18 months, but not at 1 year following surgery. (In this case, steroid therapy was tapered down 6 months after surgery and discontinued 12 months after surgery.) Normal dexamethasone suppressibility was also present when tested 18 months postoperatively. A patient reported by Lagerquist et al. (1974) had normal dexamethasone suppressibility and circadian periodicity when tested 8 months postoperatively. Two of three patients studied by Boyar et al. (1979) showed return of normal circadian periodicity when studied 8 months and 10 months postsurgery: In the first instance, this was 2 months after discontinuance of replacement therapy, and the time of discontinuance of replacement therapy was not given for the second patient. A third patient, although showing normalization of 24-h mean cortisol concentrations and resolution of the clinical features of Cushing's syndrome, had absence of circadian periodicity 11 months after surgery, as well as a subnormal responsiveness to metyrapone in studies 2 months after discontinuance of cortisol therapy. The two patients showing normalization of circadian cortisol rhythms maintained remission 1 and 2 years after surgery, respectively. Kuwayama et al. (1980) have reported absent periodicity in four of ten patients studied 6 months postoperatively. Four of nine patients studied by Bigos et al. (1980) had normal circadian periodicity. It should be noted, however, that the only study in which detailed studies were performed over a 24-h period utilizing frequent sampling was that of Boyar et al. (1979). That of Schnall et al. (1978) was based on only three time points over 24 h, and that of Bigos (1980) on only two. The nature of sampling was not specified in Kuwayamas's study (1980) and, in that of Lagerquist (1974), although more frequent sampling was performed, it was not done over a major portion of the 24-h cycle.

These postoperative findings raise questions as to the primary etiological or pathological locus in Cushing's disease. The findings of postoperative adrenocortical insufficiency indicate that, at least at that time, there was certainly no evidence of hyperfunction of remaining pituitary tissue. Such insufficiency may represent suppression of normal pituitary ACTH cells by the hypersecreting adenoma (i.e., similar to suppression of remaining adrenal cortical cells by an adrenal adenoma) or an indication of altered functional capacity of cells as an expression of the morphological alterations classified as Crooke's changes (which occur in the majority of corticotrophs in both endogenous and exogenous hypercortisolism). The presence of normal circadian periodicity in 14 of 24 postoperative patients and the normal dexamethasone suppressibility noted in two patients suggest that there had been restoration of normal CNS-pituitary interactions. This would imply a primarily pituitary etiology in such cases.

These observations should be tempered by the reports of recurrences after surgically induced remission, as well as by some of the pathological findings reported that indicate the presence of coexisting hyperplasia and adenoma, which might indicate a hypothalamic etiology for pituitary stimulation. Several cases of such recurrence have been reported anecdotally, and reference has already been made to the two cases reported by Bigos et al. (1980). Pont and Gutierrez-Hartman (1979) also reported a case that exhibited marked clinical and laboratory evidence of remission, including normal dexamethasone suppressibility and a normal cortisol response to insulin-induced hypoglycemia, with, however, recurrence of symptomatology and evidence of glucocorticoid hypersecretion 10 months postoperatively.

Such recurrences may be secondary to the pathological findings reported in other series in which more extensive hypophysectomy, rather than micro-adenomectomy, has been performed (see Chap. 6). Ludecke et al. (1976) reported that in 15 cases of Cushing's disease in which total hypophysectomy was performed, adenomas were present in 11 instances, while in four either nodular or diffuse ACTH cell hyperplasia of the anterior lobe was present. In nine of the cases with adenoma, there was also associated evidence of either diffuse or nodular ACTH cell hyperplasia. In another five patients with Nelson's syndrome in whom selective adenomectomy was performed, histological studies were reported only on two patients in whom nodular ACTH cell hyperplasia was also present in addition to adenoma. In a series reported by Carmalt et al. (1976) in which partial hypophysectomy was performed in 13 patients, four showed only focal hyperplasia of the basophils, in one there was no obvious pathology, another showed only hyalinized basophils (i.e.,

Crooke's changes), and seven had adenomata. Of the 12 survivors, 11 were in complete remission, although six of these apparently required corticosteroid replacement therapy, one of these being a patient in whom only ACTH cell hyperplasia had been noted. The second patient with hyperplasia was apparently cured by the operative procedure as of 2 years follow-up. The third patient, with hyperplasia, succumbed 4 years postsurgery and the pituitary was described as showing a *normal* pars anterior surrounded by a thick fibrous capsule. The most recent case is one reported by Lamberts et al. (1980) in which no remission was seen following removal of a 3-mm adenoma and in whom examination of the surrounding normal pituitary tissue, removed surgically, revealed multiple small masses of adenomatous basophilic cells. It is possible, therefore, that when there is an element of ACTH cell hyperplasia present in some of the patients reported to be cured by adenomectomy, over a sufficiently long time course such cells will receive sufficient hypothalamic stimulation to result in adenoma and to again present evidence of Cushing's disease. There is no way of knowing how long such stimulation (if present) has to exist before anatomical and clinical expression of disease, so at present it is difficult to say what would constitute an adequate follow-up period. If such recurrences continue to be reported, other reported findings that some patients successfully operated on have apparent normalization of CNS-pituitary function may well indicate that there are two subgroups of this disease, with either pituitary or CNS etiology.

## V. Medical Treatment

In view of the large body of experimental evidence indicating involvement of multiple neurotransmitters in the regulation of ACTH secretion (Krieger 1973) (see Chap. 2), the large body of evidence implicating serotonin as an excitatory neurotransmitter in this regard (Krieger 1978), and the experimental evidence of CNS pathophysiology in Cushing's disease (see Chap. 6), our laboratory has elected to investigate the use of antiserotonergic agents in the treatment of Cushing's disease (Krieger 1975). The available evidence indicates that serotonin acts via a hypothalamic locus of action in the stimulation of ACTH release, although there may be some effects at a pituitary level. It has also been demonstrated that cyproheptadine, which has antiserotoninergic effects (in addition to lesser effects on other neurotransmitters), inhibits both acetylcholine- and serotonin-induced release of CRF without interfering with the ability of CRF to release ACTH (Jones et al. 1979).

Studies to date indicate that in adult patients this drug appears to be effective in approximately 50% of cases (Krieger 1980). Additional published reports other than those reported from our laboratory are Barnes et al. (1977) and Marek et al. (1977). Administration of 24 mg daily is associated with a sustained clinical and laboratory remission after 2–3 months which is usually maintained with continued medication. In addition to normalization of cortisol secretion, there is also return of normal dexamethasone suppressibility and of normal corticosteroid and ACTH circadian periodicity. The longest treatment period to date has been 18 months. The side effects of hyperphagia and somnolence noted initially usually disappear spontaneously with continuation of medication. Relapses almost always occur after discontinuance of treatment. In a small number of patients, relapses may occur while on medication after successful treatment for up to 15 months. We have observed apparently permanent remission that has persisted 2.5 years following discontinuance of cyproheptadine therapy in a patient with Cushing's disease who subsequently became pregnant, delivered normally, and has no signs of active disease.

The major negative report on the efficacy of cyproheptadine was one in which five adult patients were studied (Tyrrell et al. 1976) utilizing treatment with less than the suggested dose, and with three of these patients receiving the drug for a period of 1 month or less. This drug also appears to be less effective in children (d'Ercole 1977), although here, again, therapy was for less than 1 month. There is, however, a report of complete clinical remission, in a 14-year-old boy, that was maintained after discontinuing cyproheptadine therapy after 18 months of treatment, associated with a pronounced acceleration of growth and bone maturation and remission of hypertension (Grant and Atherden 1979).

Cyproheptadine therapy is also effective in Nelson's syndrome (Krieger and Luria 1976; Hartwig et al. 1976), though no effect was noted in three patients reported by Cassar et al. (1976). In our study, we observed marked decreases in both plasma ACTH and LPH concentrations and skin pigmentation in 50% of such patients. Similar to effects in patients with Cushing's disease, remission is associated with the reappearance of normal ACTH circadian periodicity and relapse occurs after discontinuance of medication, except one instance of remission over an 18-month follow-up period after drug discontinuance (Aronin and Krieger 1980). Hartwig et al. (1976) also observed associated correction of a small visual field defect, suggesting actual tumor shrinkage similar to what has been reported in some cases of prolactin-secreting adenoma treated with bromocryptine.

In those instances of Cushing's disease where relapses occur during medication or where an unsatisfactory response to cyproheptadine has been obtained, we have noted that the use of cyproheptadine therapy together with pituitary irradiation (cobalt, 4500 rad) achieves normalization of urinary corticosteroids within the 4-week period of radiotherapy, and that it is possible to discontinue cyproheptadine within 4 months after the onset of such irradiation and achieve a permanent remission, in contrast to the period of 1 year or more usually required before remission is achieved in patients receiving cobalt irradiation alone.

There have been some surprising reports suggesting at least partial efficacy of cyproheptadine in Cushing's disease associated with ectopic tumors. One was a case of thymoma (carcinoid type) in which, after 9 weeks of response to cyproheptadine therapy, rapid clinical deterioration occurred (Doyle and O'Donovan 1977). In another case of carcinoid tumor reported by Leveston et al. (1978), cyproheptadine administration induced a clinical and laboratory remission in an 18-year-old man with gigantism and explosive Cushing's syndrome (ACTH 4200 pg/ml). It was subsequently demonstrated that growth hormone-releasing factor-like material was present in the carcinoid tumor. It might be postulated that the tumor also contained CRF-like material and that cyproheptadine was acting at this locus rather than directly on possible ACTH production by the tumor.

Metergoline has also been employed as a more specific antiserotonergic agent than cyproheptadine. There have been two reports of effective treatment of childhood Cushing's disease with this drug. In one report (Soyka 1979), remission and a normal growth pattern were observed following the onset of therapy, in marked contrast to the absence of linear growth during a 2-year period preceding treatment. In the other (Ferrari et al. 1977), laboratory response was seen within 1 week after onset of therapy, with a return to normal dexamethasone responsiveness.

As noted in Chap. 2, there are conflicting data on the role of catecholamines in modulating the secretion of ACTH. Those studies which do suggest an inhibitory role in the central regulation of CRF implicate norepinephrine as the neurotransmitter involved (Ganong 1977). Dopamine does not affect CRF release in vitro (Hillhouse et al. 1975). Acute administration of bromocryptine, however, was shown to suppress ACTH and cortisol levels in some patients with Cushing's disease and Nelson's syndrome (Lamberts et al. 1980), although no such effects were observed in another series of patients who had prior adrenalectomy (O'Mullane et al. 1978). The most detailed study of chronic treatment (Lamberts et al. 1980) indicates escape in two of five responding patients after 2–6 weeks of therapy.

Concerning reserpine, it has been claimed that long-term administration of this drug combined with pituitary irradiation is effective in inducing a remission in Cushing's disease, in contrast to only a partial response to reserpine alone (Miura et al. 1975). It is difficult to ascertain what role reserpine played, however, over and above the effect of pituitary irradiation.

At present there is still a question as to the role of neuropharmacological therapy in the treatment of Cushing's disease. This may be resolved with further follow-up of surgically and medically treated patients, and when other neuropharmacological agents are developed. If therapy directed at a pituitary or hypothalamic site is effective, this should prevent the development of Nelson's syndrome. The problems of medical therapy with regard to the need for continued drug maintenance, as well as occasional relapse during therapy, may signify that neuropharmacological therapy, specifically cyproheptadine, may be indicated as conjunctive therapy with pituitary irradiation, or as preparation for pituitary surgery should long-term studies of the latter indicate lack of significant recurrence.

Table 8.2 summarizes the considerations of available therapy in Cushing's disease. A few specific comments may be in order. In those patients with severe symptoms and signs of Cushing's disease, it is necessary to utilize therapy which will be rapidly effective. Of all the forms of therapy available, pituitary surgery (microadenomectomy) would be the choice, since it does not have the inherent disadvantages of adrenalectomy. Although one would think that rapidly effective therapy would also be indicated for children, in whom one of the major deleterious effects is stunted growth occasioned by excess corticoids, the risk of compromise of residual pituitary function by surgery in such patients, and the perhaps even greater efficacy of pituitary irradiation in this age group, would appear to make this the treatment of choice. A question has been raised with regard to the rare development of CNS tumors or hypothalamic dysfunction following irradiation of CNS leukemia or naso-

**Table 8.2.** Summary of available therapy in Cushing's disease

| | Positive aspects | Negative aspects | Specific indications |
|---|---|---|---|
| 1. Neuropharmacologic agents | No major side effects<br>No adverse effect on other pituitary functions | Not permanent cure<br>Only ca. 50% effective | Moderate disease<br>Adjunct to pituitary irradiation or surgery |
| | Prevents progression of Nelson's syndrome | Weight gain | |
| 2. Pituitary surgery | Cure if lesion 1° a pituitary one | Operative morbidity (ca. 2–5%) | Need for rapid response in severe disease |
| | | Possibility of ↓ pituitary function postoperatively<br>Occasional problems of tumor identification at surgery<br>Follow-up results recurrences<br>Rare cases where ectopic ACTH tumor discovered subsequently | Nelson's syndrome with obvious sellar enlargement |
| 3. Irradiation | No major side effects | Effective 50–80% | |
| | Usually no adverse effect on other pituitary functions (normal reproductive function posttreatment) | May have relapse (?) | |
| | Proton beam 27%, ↓ other pituitary function | Effective 89% | Moderate disease in children |
| 4. Adrenalectomy surgical | Rapid | Need for replacement therapy<br>Development of pituitary tumor (10–15%)<br>Residual adrenal tissue (ca. 5%) | |
| Medical | | Frequent escape (except for o,p'DDD)<br>Need for replacement therapy<br>Undesirable side effects | Adjunct to pituitary irradiation or surgery |

pharyngeal tumors, especially in young children. There is no large series of children irradiated for Cushing's disease with long enough follow-up to adequately assess this possibility.

In cases of moderate disease in adults, available options are pituitary irradiation, medical therapy (o,p'DDD or cyproheptadine), or pituitary surgery as discussed here.

Treatment for Nelson's syndrome should be considered in the same manner as Cushing's disease. Although it had been suggested that pituitary tumors associated with Cushing's disease are invasive and generally carry a poor prognosis (Rovit and Duane 1969; Welbourn 1969), the recent survey by Moore et al. (1976) failed to substantiate such a suggestion. In nine patients with documented pituitary enlargement in Nelson's disease, seven were alive and clinically stable an average of 10 years after pituitary tumors were discovered.

The etiology and therapy of Cushing's disease have been a subject of debate since the initial description of this disease almost 50 years ago. Recent advances in neuroendocrine physiology, endocrine assay techniques, neurosurgery, and immunocytochemistry have brought about new concepts of the pathophysiology of the disease, and may suggest subsets of etiologies with common clinical manifestations. It is inevitable that progress in all of these fields and others in the next 5 decades will further necessitate revision of present-day concepts, providing further understanding of a condition which, although rare, has served as a major stimulus for investigation of the CNS-pituitary-adrenal axis.

## References


Aronin N, Krieger DT (1980) Persistent remission of Nelson's syndrome following discontinuance of cyproheptadine treatment. N Engl J Med 302:453–455

Barnes P, Shaw K, Ross E (1977) Cushing's disease: Successful treatment with cyproheptadine. Lancet II:1148–1149

Barzilai D, Dickstein G, Kanter Y, Plavnick Y, Schramek A (1980) Complete remission of Cushing's disease by total bilateral adrenalectomy and adrenal autotransplantation. J Clin Endocrinol Metab 50:853–856

Becker D, Schumacher OP (1975) o,p'DDD therapy in invasive adrenocortical carcinoma. Ann Intern Med 82:677–679

Bennett AH, Cain JP, Dluhy RG, Tynes WV, Harrison JH, Thorn GW (1973) Surgical treatment of adrenocortical hyperplasia: 20-Year experience. J Urol 109:321–324

Bigos ST, Somma M, Rasio E, Eastman RC, Lanthier A, Johnston HH, Hardy J (1980) Cushing's disease: Management by trans-sphenoidal pituitary microsurgery. J Clin Endocrinol Metab 50:348–354

Boyar RM, Witkin M, Carruth A, Ramsey J (1979) Circadian cortisol secretory rhythms in Cushing's disease. J Clin Endocrinol Metab 48:760–765

Burke CW, Doyle FH, Joplin GF, Arnot RN, MacErlean DP, Fraser TR (1973) Cushing's disease: Treatment by pituitary implantation of radioactive gold or yttrium seeds. Quart J Med 42:693–714

Carmalt MHB, Dalton GA, Fletcher RF, Smith WT (1977) The treatment of Cushing's disease by trans-sphenoidal hypophysectomy. Quart J Med 46:119–134

Cassar J, Mashiter K, Joplin GF (1976) Cyproheptadine in Nelson's syndrome. Lancet III:426

Child DF, Burke CW, Burley DM, Rees LH, Fraser TR (1976) Drug control of Cushing's syndrome: Combined aminoglutethimide and metyrapone therapy. Acta Endocrinol 82:330–341

Cope O, Raker JW (1955) Cushing's disease: The surgical experience in the care of 46 cases. N Engl J Med 253:165–172

D'Ercole AJ, Morris MA, Underwood LE, Van Wyk JJ, Feldman JM (1977) Treatment of Cushing's disease in childhood with cyproheptadine. J Pediatr 90:834–835

Dohan FC, Raventos A, Boucot N, Rose E (1957) Roentgen therapy in Cushing's syndrome without adrenocortical tumor. J Clin Endocrinol Metab 17:8–32

Doyle D, O'Donovan DK (1977) More on cyproheptadine in Cushing's disease. N Engl J Med 296:576

Ernest I, Ekman H (1972) Adrenalectomy in Cushing's disease. Acta Endocrinol (Suppl) 160:5–41
Ferrari C, Bertazzoni A, Ghezzi M (1977) Letter to the editor. N Engl J Med 296:576–577
Fishman LM, Liddle GW, Island DP, Fleischer N, Kuchel O (1967) Effects of aminoglutethimide on adrenal function in man. J Clin Endocrinol Metab 27:481–487
Fitzgerald PA, Tyrrell JB, Brooks RM, Forsham PH, Wilson CB (1978) Cushing's disease: Secondary adrenal insufficiency after selective removal of pituitary tumors. 60th Meeting Endocrine Soc., p 250
Ganong WF (1977) Neurotransmitters involved in ACTH secretion: Catecholamines. In: ACTH and related peptides: Structure, regulation, and action. Ann NY Acad Sci 297:509–516
Grant DB, Atherden SM (1979) Cushing's disease presenting with growth failure: Clinical remission during cyproheptadine therapy. Arch Dis Child 54:466–468
Hartwig W, Kasperlik-Zaluska A, Wilczynska J, Migdalaska B (1976) Treatment of Nelson's syndrome with cyproheptadine. N Engl J Med 295:394
Heuschele R, Lampe I (1967) Pituitary irradiation for Cushing's syndrome. Radiol Clin Biol 36:27–31
Hillhouse EW, Burden J, Jones MT (1975) The effect of various putative neurotransmitters on the release of corticotrophin-releasing hormone from the hypothalamus of the rat in vitro. 1. The effect of acetylcholine and noradrenaline. Neuroendocrinology 17:1–11
Hutter AM Jr, Kayhoe DE (1966) Adrenal cortical carcinoma: Results of treatment with o,p'DDD in 138 patients. Am J Med 41:581–592
Jeffcoate WJ, Rees LH, Tomlin S, Jones AE, Edwards CRW, Besser GM (1977) Metyrapone in long-term management of Cushing's disease. Br Med J II:215–217
Jennings AS, Liddle GW, Orth DN (1977) Results of treating childhood Cushing's disease with pituitary irradiation. N Engl J Med 297:957–962
Jones MT, Birmingham M, Gillham B, Holmes M, Smith T (1979) The effect of cyproheptadine on the release of corticotrophin-releasing factor. Clin Endocrinol 10:203–204
Kjellberg RN, Kliman B (1973) A system for therapy of pituitary tumors. In: Kohler PO, Ross GT (eds) Diagnosis and treatment of pituitary tumors. Excerpta Medica, Amsterdam; American Elsevier Publ., New York, pp 234–252
Komanicky P, Spark RF, Melby JC (1978) Treatment of Cushing's syndrome with trilostane (WIN 24,540), an inhibitor of adrenal steroid biosynthesis. J Clin Endocrinol Metab 47:1042–1051
Krieger DT (1973) Neurotransmitter regulation of ACTH release. Mt Sinai J Med NY 40:302–314
Krieger DT (1980) Cyproheptadine: Drug therapy for Cushing's disease. In: Muller EE (ed) Neuroactive drugs in endocrinology. Elsevier/North Holland, Amsterdam, pp 361–370
Krieger DT, Luria M (1976) Effectiveness of cyproheptadine in decreasing plasma ACTH concentrations in Nelson's syndrome. J Clin Endocrinol Metab 43:1179–1182
Krieger DT, Amorosa L, Linick F (1975) Cyproheptadine-induced remission of Cushing's disease. N Engl J Med 293:893–896
Kuwayama A, Kageyama N, Nakane T, Watanabe M, Kanie N (1980) Anterior pituitary function after trans-sphenoidal selective microadenomectomy in Cushing's disease. VII Int. Cong. Endocrinol., Melbourne, p 385
Lagerquist LG, Meikle AW, West DC, Tyler FH (1974) Cushing's disease with cure by resection of a pituitary adenoma: Evidence against a primary hypothalamic defect. Am J Med 57:826–830
Lamberts SWJ, Klijn JGM, de Quijada M, Timmermans HAT, Uitterlinden P, Kirkenhager JC (1980) Bromocriptine and the medical treatment of Cushing's disease. In: Muller EE (ed). Neuroactive drugs in endocrinology. Elsevier/North Holland, Amsterdam, pp 371–382
Lamberts SWJ, Stefanko SZ, de Lange SA, Fermin H, van der Vijver JCM, Weber RFA, de Jong FH (1980) Failure of clinical remission after trans-sphenoidal removal of a microadenoma in a patient with Cushing's disease: Multiple hyperplastic and adenomatous cell rests in surrounding pituitary tissue. J Clin Endocrinol Metab 50:793–795
Leveston SA, Lee Y-C, Jaffe BM, Daughaday WH (1978) Massive GH and ACTH hypersecretion associated with a metastatic carcinoid tumor. 60th Meeting Endocrine Soc., p 371 (Abstract)
Linfoot JA (1975) Heavy-ion therapy: Alpha-particle therapy of pituitary tumors. In: Linfoot JA (ed) Recent advances in the diagnosis and treatment of pituitary tumors. Raven Press, New York, pp 254–267

Lipsett MB, Hertz R, Ross GT (1963) Clinical and pathophysiologic aspects of adrenocortical carcinoma. Am J Med 35:374–383

Lubitz JA, Freeman L, Okun R (1973) Mitotane in operable adrenocortical carcinoma. JAMA. 233:1109–1112

Ludecke D, Kautzky R, Saeger W, Schrader D (1976) Selective removal of hypersecreting pituitary adenomas? An analysis of endocrine function, operative and microscopical findings in 101 cases. Acta Neurochirurg 35:27–42

Luton JP, Mahoudeau JA, Bouchard P, Thieblot P, Hautecouverture M, Simon D, Laudat MH, Touitou Y, Bricaire H (1979) Treatment of Cushing's disease by o,p'DDD: Survey of 62 cases. N Engl J Med 300:459–464

MacFarlane DA (1958) Cancer of the adrenal cortex. Ann R Coll Surg 23:155

Marek J, Matys Z, Gregorova L (1977) Cyproheptadine in Cushing's syndrome. Lancet III: 653–654

Misbin RI, Canary J, Willard D (1976) Aminoglutethimide in the treatment of Cushing's syndrome. J Clin Pharmacol 16:645–651

Miura K, Aida M, Mihara A, Kato K, Ojima M, Demura R, Demura H, Okuyama M (1975) Treatment of Cushing's disease with reserpine and pituitary irradiation. J Clin Endocrinol Metab 41:511–526

Moore TJ, Dluhy RG, Williams GH, Cain JP (1976) Nelson's syndrome: Frequency, prognosis, and effect of prior pituitary irradiation. Ann Intern Med 85:731–734

O'Mullane N, Walker B, Jefferson J, Hipkin L, Diver M, Davis C (1978) Lack of effect of bromocriptine on ACTH levels in patients with bilateral adrenalectomy for pituitary-dependent Cushing's syndrome. J Endocrinol Invest 1:355–357

Orth DN, Liddle GW (1971) Results of treatment in 108 patients with Cushing's syndrome. N Engl J Med 285:243–247

Ostuni JA, Roginsky MS (1975) Metastatic adrenal cortical carcinoma. Arch Intern Med 135:1257–1258

Plotz CM, Knowlton AI, Ragan C (1952) The natural history of Cushing's syndrome. Am J Med 13:597–614

Pont A, Gutierrez-Hartman A (1979) Cushing's disease: Recurrence after a surgically induced remission. Arch Intern Med 139:938–940

Prinz RA, Brooks MH, Lawrence AM, Paloyan E (1979) Cushing's disease: The role of adrenalectomy and autotransplantation. Surg Clin North Am 59:159–165

Rees LH, Bloomfield GA, Gilkes JJF, Jeffcoate WJ, Besser GM (1977) ACTH as a tumor marker. In: Krieger DT, Ganong WF (eds) ACTH and related peptides: Structure, regulation, and action. NY Acad Sci, New York, pp 603–620

Rovit RL, Duane TD (1969) Cushing's syndrome and pituitary tumors. Am J Med 46:416–427

Salassa RM, Laws ER Jr, Carpenter PC, Northcutt RC (1978) Trans-sphenoidal removal of pituitary microadenoma in Cushing's disease. Mayo Clin Proc 53:24–28

Schnall AM, Brodkey JS, Kaufman B, Pearson OH (1978) Pituitary function after removal of pituitary microadenomas in Cushing's disease. J Clin Endocrinol Metab 47:410–417

Scott WH Jr, Liddle GW, Mulherin JL Jr, McKenna TJ, Stroup SL, Rhamy RK (1977) Surgical experience with Cushing's disease. Ann Surg 85:524–534

Seters van AP, Jenny M, Querido A (1965) Unilateral adrenalectomy followed by pituitary irradiation in Cushing's disease: With observations on cortisol secretion after therapy. Acta Endocrinol 48:253–262

Soffer LJ, Iannaccone A, Gabrilove JL (1961) Cushing's syndrome: A study of 50 patients. Am J Med 30:129–146

Soyka L (1979) Successful trial of metergoline in juvenile Cushing's disease (abstract). Pediatr Res 13:385

Tyrrell JB, Brooks RM, Fitzgerald PA, Cofoid PB, Forsham PH, Wilson CB (1978) Selective trans-sphenoidal resection of pituitary microadenomas. N Engl J Med 298:753–758

Tyrrell JB, Brooks RM, Forsham PH (1976) More on cyproheptadine. N Engl J Med 295:1137–1138

Walter RM, Ensinck JW, Ricketts H, Kendall JW, Williams RH (1973) Insulin and ACTH production by a streptozotocin-responsive islet cell carcinoma. Am J Med 55:667–670

Welbourn RB (1966) Cushing's syndrome. Scott Med J 11:227–237

Welbourn RB, Montgomery DAD, Kennedy TL (1971) The natural history of treated Cushing's syndrome. Br J Surg 58:1–16

# Subject Index


ACTH
  action
    effect on cAMP 23, 25
    on adrenal phosphorylase 26
    on adrenal protein synthesis 25
    on adrenal size 24
    on aldosterone synthesis 26
    on cortisol metabolism 28
    on 5α-reductase 26
    on glucocorticoid synthesis 25
    on pigmentation 28
    on plasma cortisol levels 27
    on receptor 23, 25
    role of calcium 23
  anterior pituitary regulation of
    by neurotransmitters 10, 11
    effect of adrenalectomy 14
    glucocorticoid feedback 12
    neuroanatomical pathways 11
  behavioral effects of 29
  chemistry of
    precursor form 5, 7
    processing of
      anterior lobe 5, 7
      intermediate lobe 6, 40
  ectopic tumor 41
  intermediate lobe
    glucocorticoid feedback on 17
  pituitary
    in Cushing's disease 40
    in normal subjects 40
  pituitary immunocytochemistry 7
  plasma
    bioassay of 70, 82
    circadian periodicity of 14, 15, 17
    half-life of 26, 83
    levels in Cushing's disease 83, 84
    levels in Cushing's syndrome 84
    levels in Nelson's syndrome 85, 87
    levels in normal subjects 84
    metabolic clearance rate of 27
    radioimmunoassay of 82
    response to
      insulin 86
      Vasopressin 86
Adrenal adenoma 57
Adrenal carcinoma 58, 59
  Cushing's disease 57
Adrenal nodular hyperplasia 57
  laboratory tests in 101, 102
Adrenal size
  effect of ACTH 24
  growth factors 24
  neural regulation of 24
Adrenal visualization of
  angiography 112
  CAT scan 108, 109–111
  radioiodine scan 107
  ultrasonography 108, 109
  X-ray 105
α-MSH
  intermediate lobe, response to stress 17
Aminoglutethimide
  therapy of
    adrenal carcinoma 120
    Cushing's disease
    ectopic ACTH syndrome 120
APUD concept 61

β-Endorphin
  pituitary
    in Cushing's disease 41
    in normal subjects 40
  plasma concentrations of
    normal levels 16
    response to stimuli 16
β-Lipotropin
  effect of glucocorticoids on 16
  plasma concentrations of
    in Cushing's disease 87
    in Nelson's syndrome 87
    normal levels 85, 87
    response to insulin-induced hypoglycemia 86
  processing of 5, 7
  release of 16
Bromocryptine, therapy of Cushing's disease 133

Circadian periodicity of
  adrenal response to ACTH 14
  adrenal secretion 14
  CRF 15
  plasma ACTH concentrations 14, 15
  plasma cortisol
    characterization of 16

Circadian periodicity of plasma cortisol
following microadenomectomy 129
in normal subjects 15
in CNS disease 15
in Cushing's disease 46, 78–80, 101
Corticosteroid-binding globulin, nature of 76
Corticosteroids
actions on
carbohydrate metabolism 33
central nervous system 34
electrolytes 33, 47
fat metabolism 33, 47
gastric secretion 34
immune system 34
protein metabolism 33, 47
biosynthesis of 35–37, 39
feedback effects of 12
membrane effects of 38
"permissive" action of 38
receptors 13, 35
regulation of synthesis
effect of ACTH 25
effect of prostaglandins 26
Cortisol (plasma)
binding to corticosteroid-binding globulin 76
circadian periodicity of
in Cushing's disease 78–80, 101
in normal subjects 15, 16
episodic secretion of 76
levels
in Cushing's disease, Cushing's syndrome 102
in normal subjects 75, 78
methods for determination of 77
response to ACTH 27, 101
response to dexamethasone 101
response to vasopressin 101
Cortisol production rate, in normal subjects 82
Cortisol (urine)
response to ACTH 102
response to dexamethasone suppression
in Cushing's disease, Cushing's syndrome 102
in normal subjects 102
response to metyrapone 102
Cushing's disease
ACTH responsiveness 88, 101
age incidence of 57, 58
behavioral changes in 51, 66
causes of death in 48
childhood 53
clinical manifestations of 47, 49
cyclicity in 52, 63
definition of 1
dexamethasone responsiveness 91–94, 101, 102
differential diagnosis of 64–67
vs. alcoholism 64
Cushing's disease
differential diagnosis of
vs. depression 64, 65
vs. obesity 64, 65
extraocular palsy in 60
familial incidence of 53
growth hormone
circadian periodicity of 95
response to stimuli 95
hirsutism in 51
hypertension
incidence of 48
pathophysiology of 48
laboratory diagnosis of 73–104
LHRH response 94, 95
metyrapone responsiveness 90
osteoporosis in 50
pathogenesis
hypothalamic etiology 46
pituitary etiology 44, 45
periodic hormonogenesis in 52
peripheral blood findings in 34
pituitary ACTH in
concentrations of 41
forms of 40
pituitary apoplexy in 60
pituitary endorphin
concentrations of 41
pituitary LPH in 41
pituitary pathology 45, 46, 59
pituitary size in 45, 59
pituitary tumors in 60
plasma ACTH in
basal levels 85, 87
effect of somatostatin on 95
venous catheterization studies 103
plasma lipotropin in 85, 87
pregnancy in 53
prolactin levels in 95
circadian periodicity of 95
remission (spontaneous) 52
testosterone levels in 51, 96
thyroid function in 96
treatment of
adrenalectomy 56, 122–124, 134
aminoglutethimide 124
bromocryptine 133
cyproheptadine 131
metergoline 133
metyrapone 125
o, p′DDD 124
pituitary irradiation 126–127
pituitary surgery 127–131
principles of 122
TRH response 94
vasopressin responsiveness 88, 89
X-ray findings in
pituitary 45, 104, 127

Cushing's syndrome
adrenal visualization in 107, 108, 111
alcohol-induced Cushing's syndrome 65
circadian variation of plasma cortisol 100, 101
definition of 1
dexamethasone suppression test in 91, 99, 100, 101
metyrapone responsiveness 90, 99
plasma ACTH levels in 100, 101
pseudo-Cushing's syndrome 66
treatment of
adrenal adenoma 119
adrenal carcinoma 119, 120
vasopressin responsiveness 88, 99, 101
Cyproheptadine
therapy of Cushing's disease 131
combined with X-ray 131
therapy of ectopic tumors 131

Depression
differential diagnosis from Cushing's disease 100
in Cushing's disease 51
Dexamethasone suppression test
abnormal response to 93
effects of drugs on 93
in alcohol-induced "pseudo-Cushing's" 67
multiple-dose test
high dose test
in Cushing's disease 91, 101
in Cushing's syndrome 91, 101
normal response 91, 101
low dose test
in Cushing's disease 91, 99, 101
following microadenomectomy 129
in Cushing's syndrome 91, 99, 101
normal response 91, 99, 101

Ectopic ACTH-producing tumors
ACTH concentrations in 41, 95, 97, 100
ACTH, nature of 41, 42, 62
ACTH responsiveness 101
β-endorphin in 42
β-LPH in 42, 85, 87
β-MSH in 42
circadian variation of plasma ACTH 101
clinical course of 62
criteria for ectopic hormone production 61, 62
dexamethasone suppression testing in 91, 100–102
γ-MSH in 42
metyrapone test in 100, 102
other hormones in 64
sex incidence of 62
treatment of 120
types of tumors 61, 62
vasopressin test in 64, 101
venous catheterization studies in 103

γ-Lipotropin
pituitary
Cushing's disease 41
normal 40
plasma
normal levels 86
response to insulin-induced hypoglycemia 86
response to Pitressin 86
Growth hormone
circadian periodicity of 47, 95
responsiveness to testing 95

Hyperpigmentation
in Cushing's disease 51, 60
in ectopic ACTH syndrome 62
Hypophysectomy
complications of 128
cure rate of 128
effect on laboratory parameters 129
recurrences following 130
treatment for Cushing's disease 127–130, 134
Hypothalamus, pathology in Cushing's disease 45

Insulin tolerance test
in Cushing's disease, Cushing's syndrome 90, 91
in normal subjects 86
response of plasma ACTH 16
response of plasma β-LPH 16
response of plasma endorphin 16
Irradiation therapy 126, 127, 131

17-Ketosteroids (urine) 81
Cushing's disease, Cushing's syndrome, levels in 102
normal levels 102

LHRH test in Cushing's disease 94, 95

Melanocyte-stimulating hormone (MSH)
α-MSH 6
β-MSH 6
γ-MSH
chemistry of 6
in ectopic tumors 42
Metergoline, therapy of Cushing's disease 133
Metyrapone test
overnight test 89
rationale of testing 89
response in Cushing's disease 90, 99, 102
response in Cushing's syndrome 90, 99, 100, 102

Metyrapone test
  response in normal subjects 90, 102
  response of plasma endorphin 16
Metyrapone
  treatment of Cushing's disease 125

Nelson's syndrome
  clinical characterization 55
  gonadal tumors in 56
  pigmentation in 56
  pituitary X-ray in 56
  plasma ACTH in 85, 87
  plasma LPH in 87
  sex incidence of 56
  treatment of 135

Obesity, differential diagnosis from Cushing's disease 65
17-OHCS (urine), normal levels 75
o, p'DDD
  therapy of
    adrenal carcinoma 119
    Cushing's disease 124
    ectopic ACTH syndrome 120
Osteoporosis 50

Pathology
  adrenal, in Cushing's disease 57
  pituitary
    in Cushing's disease 45, 46, 59, 60

Pituitary, intermediate lobe
  ACTH processing in 7
Pregnancy in Cushing's disease 53
Prolactin, circadian periodicity of 47, 95

Reserpine, therapy of Cushing's disease 133

Testosterone levels in Cushing's disease
  female 51
  male 51
TRH test in Cushing's disease 94
Trilostane, therapy of Cushing's disease 126

Vasopressin
  as CRF 9
  in ectopic ACTH syndrome 64
  response of β-LPH to 16
  response of plasma ACTH to 16
  response of plasma cortisol
    in Cushing's disease 88, 89, 101
    in Cushing's syndrome 101
    in ectopic ACTH syndrome 101

X-ray findings
  of adrenal 105, 107
  of pituitary
    Addison's disease 54
    Cushing's disease 45, 56, 104–107
    Nelson's syndrome 54, 56, 104, 106

MIX
Papier aus verantwortungsvollen Quellen
Paper from responsible sources
FSC® C105338

If you have any concerns about our products,
you can contact us on
**ProductSafety@springernature.com**

In case Publisher is established outside the EU,
the EU authorized representative is:
**Springer Nature Customer Service Center GmbH**
**Europaplatz 3, 69115 Heidelberg, Germany**

Printed by Libri Plureos GmbH
in Hamburg, Germany